THE
FIBER
PRIMER

THE NO NONSENSE LIBRARY

NO NONSENSE HEALTH GUIDES

Women's Health and Fitness
A Diet for Lifetime Health
A Guide to Exercise and Fitness Equipment
How to Tone and Trim Your Trouble Spots
Stretch for Health
Unstress Your Life
Calories, Carbohydrates and Sodium
Permanent Weight Loss
All about Vitamins and Minerals
Your Emotional Health and Well-Being
Reducing Cholesterol
Lower Your Blood Pressure
Soothe Your Aches and Pains
Walk for Health

NO NONSENSE FINANCIAL GUIDES

NO NONSENSE REAL ESTATE GUIDES

NO NONSENSE LEGAL GUIDES

NO NONSENSE CAREER GUIDES

NO NONSENSE SUCCESS GUIDES

NO NONSENSE COOKING GUIDES

NO NONSENSE WINE GUIDES

NO NONSENSE PARENTING GUIDES

NO NONSENSE STUDENT GUIDES

NO NONSENSE AUTOMOTIVE GUIDES

NO NONSENSE PHOTOGRAPHY GUIDES

NO NONSENSE GARDENING GUIDES

NO NONSENSE HEALTH GUIDE®

THE FIBER PRIMER

How to Build a Diet High in the Health Power of Fiber

By the Editors of *PREVENTION* Magazine

Longmeadow Press

Notice

This book is intended as a reference volume only, not as a medical manual or guide to self-treatment. It is not intended as a substitute for the medical advice of physicians. The reader should regularly consult a physician in general, and particularly for any symptoms. If you suspect that you have a medical problem, we urge you to seek competent medical help. Keep in mind that exercise and nutritional needs vary from person to person, depending on age, sex, health status, and individual variations. The information here is intended to help you make informed decisions about your health, not as a substitute for any treatment that may have been prescribed by your doctor.

The Fiber Primer

Library of Congress Cataloging-in-Publication Data

The Fiber primer : how to build a diet high in the health power of fiber / by the editors of Prevention magazine.
     p.   cm. — (No nonsense health guide)
  ISBN 0-681-41021-6 paperback
  1. High-fiber diet—Recipes.   I. Prevention (Emmaus, Pa.)
II. Series: No-nonsense health guide.
RM237.6.F55 1991
613.2'6—dc20   90–25654
                                              CIP

Compiled and edited by Marcia Holman

Book design by Rodale Design Staff

Photographs by Carl Doney, p. 85; John P. Hamel, p. 37; Mitch Mandel, pp. 10, 28, 43; Rodale Stock Images, pp. 19, 50, 76, 86; Sally Shenk Ullman, p. 85.

Printed in the United States of America on acid-free paper ∞

0 9 8 7 6 5 4 3 2 1   paperback

Contents

How to Make Sense of Fiber

Fiber has become fashionable.

Once regarded as roughage—"nature's scouring pad," whose main function was to clean out your system—dietary fiber has gained new respect—and a new face. Doctors sing the praises of a fiber-rich diet; food manufacturers scramble to include fiber in more and more products.

What this means is that you no longer have to spoon through a bland bowl of porridge or gnaw on a grainy bread that tastes like wood shavings to get your fair share of fiber. You can, for example, choose among a dazzling array of cereals, breads, or even snack cakes that are brimming with bran, be it wheat, oat, rice, or corn bran.

Is fiber worthy of all the fanfare? You bet. There are now impressive scientific studies that have found that fiber plays an important role in protecting us from ills ranging from the merely annoying to the truly life threatening. Fiber, researchers found, can help prevent and/or provide some relief from constipation, hemorrhoids, diverticulosis (an intestinal disorder), heart disease, diabetes, and even colon cancer. One notable Dutch study followed 871 middle-aged men for ten years and found that men with a low intake of dietary fiber had a risk of death from all causes three times higher than that of men with a high intake. The researchers concluded that "a diet containing at least 37 grams of dietary fiber per day may be protective against chronic diseases in Western societies."

What the scientists discovered is that fiber comes in not one but several forms, and that it doesn't just pass through your body but plays a healing part within your body. The insoluble form of fiber found mainly in grains, for example, adds bulk to the diet and relieves constipation. This fiber also speeds up the digestive process, possibly minimizing exposure to harmful wastes in the intestinal tract, which means protection against colon cancer. Soluble fiber, abundant in oat bran, beans, and many fruits and vegetables, may bind to cholesterol and flush it from the body, which in the long run means lower risk of heart disease. This fiber has also been shown to slow the release of sugars into the bloodstream, which is a boon for diabetics.

Perhaps one of the more intriguing findings is that fiber can be an effective diet aid. High-fiber foods make you feel full longer so you won't binge. Also, calories from high-fiber foods count less (they're escorted through your body more quickly) and are less likely to be stored as fat than calories from fat are.

Despite these persuasive findings and the fact that fiber is relatively easy to obtain (it naturally abounds in everything from barley to blueberries and prunes to pinto beans), you may not be getting enough fiber to do you much good. If you are like most Americans, you're probably consuming about 15 grams of fiber a day—roughly half the protective amount.

What's more, you may be utterly confused as to exactly how to bulk up your diet for the most health benefits.

The Fiber Primer gives you the ABCs of fiber. You'll learn about the five forms of fiber, which foods pack the highest fiber punch, and how to use fiber to relieve constipation, lower your cholesterol, lose weight, protect you from diabetes and heart disease, and generally bulk up your health.

A Get-Acquainted Guide to Fiber

We are living, as one nutritional researcher put it, in the era of the "fiber fuss."

Not since Sylvester Graham campaigned for the revival of whole wheat bread in the 1830s has there been so much energy and attention focused on the mainly undigestible portion of the foods we eat—the bran of grains, the pulp of fruit, the crunchy cell walls of vegetables, and the squishiness of beans. In other words, the fiber.

Nor have food makers ever shown such an interest in adding more fiber to their products. Having watched the surge in popularity of high-fiber breakfast cereals, food makers are eager to fortify other foods with fiber in hopes of appealing to an increasingly fiber-conscious public.

But the question remains: Why all the fuss?

Because, in the maintenance of good health, fiber plays a role that is even larger than hype. There is now solid scientific evidence to show that fiber is an antidote for many of the chronic illnesses that plague us today.

1

Those illnesses range in severity from hemorrhoids to heart disease, and fiber helps prevent them in several ways. It adds bulk to the diet and relieves constipation, it binds to cholesterol and flushes it from the body, and it speeds up the digestion process, minimizing our exposure to potentially harmful waste products in the intestinal tract.

Indeed, we know now that fiber isn't just roughage, whose main benefit, it was once thought, was to clean out the system much as a scouring pad scrubs out a pot.

In fact, fiber isn't even one substance but many different kinds of substances. And the more you know about the many ways fiber can help you, the more you'll want to include fiber-rich foods as an integral part of your overall health plan.

The Many Faces of Fiber

Dietary fiber is found only in plant foods—whole grains, fruits, and vegetables—and has certain identifiable traits. It absorbs water to one degree or another as it moves through the digestive system. But unlike other dietary substances like protein, fat, and most starch, it remains undigested for much or all of the trip. It passes through the small intestine and enters the colon virtually intact.

The different ways fiber behaves in your body.   Not all fiber is created equal. There are two main types—insoluble (which, for the most part, remains undigested) and soluble (which is eventually almost totally digested in the large intestine).

If you are interested in raising your fiber intake in order to prevent illness, keep in mind that each of the two fibers plays a different role in your health. One type of fiber might be great for one type of health problem but not affect another health problem at all.

Wheat bran, for instance, is effective in relieving constipation and possibly the diseases related to constipation.

On the other hand, pectin, a type of soluble fiber found in apples, oranges, and other produce as well as dried beans, chickpeas, and oat bran, can help lower cholesterol levels; wheat bran may not.

Pectin and oat bran can also help diabetics control their blood sugar levels.

For the best health benefits, it is important that you get both kinds of fiber. Fortunately, many high-fiber foods contain both kinds of fiber.

Insoluble Fiber: What It Can Do For You

Crunchy and crisp, insoluble fiber is found in the woody stalks, stems, peels, and skins of fruits and vegetables and in the bran (the seedcoat) of whole grains.

Scientists have identified cellulose, hemicellulose (no relation), and lignin as the three plant components most loaded with insoluble fiber. These components absorb water as they move through the digestive tract and stay fairly intact from start to finish—during the period that fiber experts call "transit time." The result: an increase in stool bulk and a faster journey through your system. The keep-moving style of insoluble fiber makes it a natural hedge for a number of intestinal-related disorders.

Hemorrhoid helper. Itching, bleeding, and pain are some of the unpleasant but all-too-common symptoms of hemorrhoids, which seem to be the curse of the civilized world. It's an undiscriminating affliction—athletes get them, pregnant women get them, and so does half of the entire population over age 50.

Eating high-fiber foods helps to form soft stools that can be passed regularly, without strain and pain. And regular, easy bowel movements save wear and tear on existing hemorrhoids and prevent hemorrhoids from forming in the first place. Fiber pushes waste out of the bowel before it forms hard, unmanageable stools that cause or inflame hemorrhoids.

When people with hemorrhoids bulk up on bran, studies show, they experience less pain and bleeding with bowel movements. Danish doctors treated 51 hemorrhoid sufferers with either a fiber supplement or a look-alike placebo. After six weeks, the people who took the fiber supplement had better bowel movements and suffered far less pain and bleeding than those who did not increase their fiber intake.

"A lifetime history of a high-fiber diet is the best way to prevent hemorrhoids, and switching to a high-fiber diet is also the best way to treat many types," says Melvin Bubrick, M.D., a surgeon at Park Nicollet Medical Center in Minneapolis, Minnesota.

"People usually feel better within three or four days after starting a high-fiber diet, but it might take them as long as two weeks to adjust to the new diet," he says.

One way to defeat diverticulosis.   Thousands of Americans over age 50 are walking around with this disease without knowing it. It is possibly due to increased pressure created in the bowel by constipation, causing little pouches to poke through the intestinal wall like bubbles through a punctured tire. These pouches are called diverticuli. Usually they go unnoticed. But should the outpouchings become inflamed—as they do easily—you have diverticulitis. Blood vessels can burst and bleed. And after years of strain, the intestinal muscles can stiffen, trapping the stools. At that point, you need to be hosptialized to have your septic system cleaned out.

Too little fiber is what causes the disease. Without fiber, stools petrify and become stranded in the bowel.

On the other hand, researchers found that a high-fiber diet can relieve more than 90 percent of the symptoms of diverticular disease. In a British study, 75 people with diverticular disease were treated with a high-fiber diet. Over 90 percent remained symptom-free for five to seven years.

Apparently dietary fiber absorbs water like a sponge and molds waste products into soft stools that can be passed along quickly and effortlessly.

If you want to keep your system regular, experts suggest you start by adding up to 2 tablespoons of bran a day to your cereal, hamburger patties, meat loaf, muffins, casseroles, even your fruit juice. Look for coarse bran varieties. Nutritionists at Cornell University showed that coarsely ground wheat bran holds more water in the feces and speeds stools along more rapidly than fine bran.

Counteracting colon cancer.   Colorectal (large bowel) or colon cancer is thought to be triggered by the presence of carcinogens in the digestive tract. Sometimes the carcinogens are present in foods, and sometimes they're produced by intestinal bacteria. Either way, the bulking action of insoluble fiber may empty the colon faster, flushing out the carcinogens before the body can absorb them. Insoluble fiber may also change the environment of the intestinal tract, thereby reducing the production of carcinogens, which can occur in normal digestion.

For these reasons, fiber is now considered one of the leading dietary weapons, if not *the* leading weapon, in the war against colon cancer. ''We feel pretty confident that fiber is involved in the prevention of colon cancer,'' says Joseph Cullen, Ph.D., of the National Cancer Institute's Division of Cancer Prevention and Control. ''It appears that people who eat more fiber have more protection against colon cancer.''

Of all the fibers, wheat bran seems to be the most effective fiber against colon cancer. To work wheat bran into your diet, choose cereals, pasta, and breads that have not been refined and that are made with whole wheat versus wheat flour. Wheat bread, for instance, isn't necessarily high in fiber.

Soluble Fiber for Super Health

Bite into a ripe, juicy pear. You've just sampled the kind of fiber that doesn't seem like fiber. Unlike its stalwart, insoluble counterpart, soluble fiber is virtually all digested, so it lacks the valuable bulking abilities of insoluble fiber. But before it's broken down, soluble fiber forms a kind of gel as it absorbs water in the intestinal tract.

Probably because of this odd characteristic, soluble fibers such as pectin and gums tend to slow down the body's digestion of food. And this digestion slowdown can benefit your body in several ways.

A diabetes fighter.   Not long ago, many adult diabetics resigned themselves to a life of chronic obesity and daily insulin injections. But some doctors are now using high-fiber diets to reduce diabetic patients' weight and their insulin needs.

''Many diabetics don't need insulin. They need a diet program,'' says James W. Anderson, M.D., of the University of Kentucky College of Medicine in Lexington, who is a recognized pioneer in the field of dietary fiber. "With intensive diet therapy, the majority of diabetic patients can go off insulin."

Using a high-fiber, ultra-low-fat diet, Dr. Anderson claims that he has been able to reduce the insulin needs of his patients anywhere from 25 to 100 percent, depending on the type of diabetes.

In one experiment conducted by Dr. Anderson, 20 adult-onset diabetics were fed the standard low-carbohydrate diet for about a week, during which time their insulin doses averaged 26 units a day. Then they switched to a diet high in carbohydrates and fiber. On the high-carbohydrate, high-fiber diet there was a rapid drop in insulin requirements. Insulin shots could be completely discontinued in eight patients, says Dr. Anderson.

Why does a diet rich in complex carbohydrates and fiber work so well? First, complex carbohydrates take longer to break down into glucose. And according to Dr. Anderson, the soluble fiber—particularly the kind found in dried beans, oat bran, and barley—slows that breakdown even more.

"After you eat a meal, there is a big pulse of carbohydrates entering the system," he says. "Fiber slows the absorption so there is a gradual release of it into the body."

Other scientists have added fiber supplements to otherwise normal diets and recorded significantly lower blood sugar and reduced need for insulin. But Dr. Anderson contends that the best results are obtained when the patient's entire diet is altered.

A hedge against heart disease.   High cholesterol levels are one of the primary causes of heart disease; and soluble fiber, along with exercise and low-fat foods, seems to bring cholesterol levels tumbling down.

Many studies have been conducted to test the effect of soluble fiber on both normal subjects and those with high cholesterol levels. Reviewing the results, one expert concluded that for the most part, soluble fiber lowers LDL (the low-density lipoprotein or "bad" cholesterol) levels without significantly decreasing the level of HDL (the high-density lipoprotein dubbed the "good" kind of cholesterol that is correlated with a decrease in heart disease).

Fiber also acts quickly. In a study by Dr. Anderson, volunteers with cholesterol counts in the caution zone—up around 260 milligrams per deciliter—experienced a 20 percent reduction in cholesterol levels in only 11 days. All they did was add either of two fiber sources—oat bran or beans—to their daily diet. Otherwise they didn't change their diet at all.

Counterpunch high cholesterol.   Pectin—the gummy substance that helps to hold the plant cell walls together and is found in most vegetables and fruits, especially in the flesh of the apple or the stringy membranes of citrus sections—might be the best protection of all against cholesterol-related problems.

True vegetarians have unusually low cholesterol levels because of the large amount of pectin in their diets, according to David Kirtchevsky, Ph.D., of the Wistar Institute in Philadelphia.

Some researchers say that these pectin-type fibers capture excess cholesterol in the digestive tract and flush it out of the body before it can be reabsorbed. Others say that fiber selectively raises the level of HDL cholesterol.

Defend yourself from gallstone formation.   A buildup of cholesterol in the bile can contribute to painful gallstones in the gallbladder. Studies have shown that fiber may play a great part in preventing gallstones from forming. Researchers in Italy studied gallstone formation in 320 people and found that half of the people who later developed gallstones ate less vegetable and fruit fiber than the people who were free from gallstone formation.

Fiber Fights Flab

One health benefit the two types of fiber share is their ability to help you control weight. Fiber has been referred to as "nature's natural brake on eating too much."

High-fiber soluble and insoluble foods—fruits and grains—satisfy the appetite while adding very few calories to the meal. Put another way, fiber fills you up but not out.

Studies have shown that people lose weight when they eat more fiber, even when they don't go out of their way to change

Finding the Fiber You Need

The different types of fiber play different health roles in your body. Some fibers are better for protecting your heart, while others help counteract constipation. For optimum health benefits, choose a variety of fiber foods.

Fiber Type	Probable Functions	Food Sources
Cellulose (I)	Relieves constipation; counteracts carcinogens in the intestinal tract; modulates glucose; curbs weight gain	Apples, bran and whole-grain cereals, brazil nuts, brussels sprouts, carrots, lima beans, peanuts, pears, peas, rhubarb, whole wheat flour and bread
Gums (S)	Lower cholesterol; modulate glucose levels	Barley, dried beans, oat bran, oatmeal, oats, psyllium, rye
Hemi-cellulose (I)	Relieves constipation; counteracts carcinogens in the intestinal tract; curbs weight gain	Apples, bananas, beets, bran and whole-grain cereals, green beans, brussels sprouts, lima beans, peas, radishes, sweet corn, whole wheat bread

their eating habits. In Sweden, for example, researchers asked a group of women weighing between 150 and 250 pounds to add a supplement of guar gum (a particular form of soluble fiber) or wheat bran (a kind of insoluble fiber) to their diet twice a day for ten weeks but not to change their diet in any other way. By the study's end, the women had lost an average of about 15 pounds each.

Fiber Type	Probable Functions	Food Sources
Lignin (I)	Escorts bile acids and cholesterol out of the intestines; offers protection against colon cancer and gallstone formation	Apples, bran and whole grain cereals, brazil nuts, cabbage, grapefruit, peaches, peanuts, pears, peas, strawberries, tomatoes, whole wheat bread
Pectin (S)	Lowers cholesterol; counters bile acids in the intestinal tract; offers protection against colon cancer and gallstone formation	Apples, bananas, beets, carrots, figs, okra, pears, plums, potatoes, strawberries

NOTE: "I" denotes insoluble fiber; "S" denotes soluble fiber.

How to Reach your Fiber Quota

Fortunately, all fiber-containing foods have both insoluble and soluble fiber in varying proportions. So if you eat lots of fiber-rich foods, you should get plenty of both types.

How much fiber is enough? Americans currently consume, on the average, between 5 and 14 grams of fiber every day.

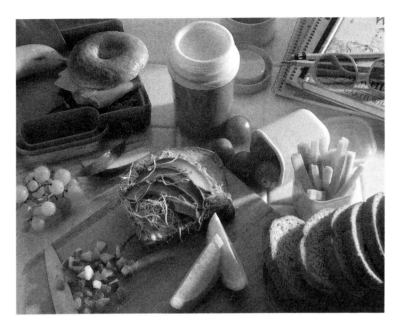

When you pack your lunch box with a good mix of foods high in insoluble and soluble fiber, you also pack health insurance. The bulk in whole-grain breads helps counter constipation and colon cancer while the soluble fiber in apples, raisins, and carrots helps control cholesterol and diabetes. And both *kinds of fiber combat obesity; they fill you up without filling you out.*

Compared to the average diet of people in many Third-World countries, that's low—too low. The National Cancer Institute recommends upping the ante to between 20 and 35 grams a day.

Double up with a good mix of fiber foods. Most Americans would be wise to merely double their fiber consumption, from an average of 15 grams to 30 grams a day. And that should come from a varied diet that includes both kinds of fiber.

In other words, don't rely on just a high-fiber cereal. It's better to divide your extra fiber into several different food sources.

"The best advice for the average person is to eat a mix of all the different kinds of fiber," says David Klurfeld, Ph.D., assistant professor at the Wistar Institute. "Eat whole-grain foods, fruits, and vegetables."

Focus on the highest-fiber foods. Refer to the tables in this chapter to help you select the top food sources that pack the most punch fiber-wise. Then review the scrumptious recipes in the chapters that follow. You'll soon discover that reaching your fiber goal is easier—and tastier—than you think.

A Word about Fiber Supplements

Eating a high-fiber diet has several advantages over taking your fiber in pill form. For starters, eating crunchy, succulent fiber-packed foods really satisfies your taste buds and tummy more than swallowing a capsule might. What's more, fiber-packed foods also tend to be chock-full of vitamins and minerals. And fiber-packed foods are very low in fat. So a shift to a fiber-rich diet is a shift to a more healthful diet overall.

Still, hectic lifestyles sometimes interfere with the best diet-wise intentions. If you find that your fiber intake consistently falls short of the recommendations given earlier, you may want to consider a fiber supplement. Here are some guidelines:

- Choose the supplements made of compressed, coarse fiber, like wheat bran or soy fiber. The ground-up husk of the psyllium seed yields a gummy fiber used to make psyllium muciloid—a bowel regulator (thanks to its insoluble-fiber component)—and is a good source of soluble fiber.
- Steer clear of powdered cellulose. Although used in some fiber supplements and in low-calorie bread, the processed cellulose (ground up and powdered) doesn't appear to work as well as when it's in the original form.
- Drink lots of fluids. Whether you get your fiber from food or from supplements, you need to increase your fluid intake to the equivalent of six to eight glasses a day. Otherwise, since insoluble fiber acts like a sponge in the intestinal tract, you risk dehydration.

Good Fiber Sources

You can mix and match foods with high, moderate, and slight amounts of fiber to boost your total fiber intake at breakfast and throughout the day. Here are some good sources to get you started.

Food	Portion	Fiber (g)
Bread		
Country oat	2 slices	6.0
Whole wheat, stone-ground	2 slices	4.5
Wheat, reduced-calorie	2 slices	4.0
Mixed grain	2 slices	3.2
Rye	2 slices	3.1
English muffin, wheat	1	3.0
Pita, whole wheat	1 pocket	2.8
Corn bread	1 piece	2.7
Cracked wheat	2 slices	2.6
Bran muffin	1	2.5
Bran oat cakes	2	2.0
Breakfast Cereals, Cold		
100% bran-type		
With added fiber	½ cup	14.0
Regular	⅓ cup	10.0
With oat bran	½ cup	8.0
Multibran	⅓ cup	6.5
Oatmeal flakes	1 cup	6.0
Corn bran, ready-to-eat	⅔ cup	5.4
40% bran-type flakes	⅔ cup	5.3
Bran-type flakes with raisins	1 oz.	5.0
Oat bran, crunchy types	1 oz.	5.0
Bran squares	⅔ cup	4.6
Breakfast Cereals, Hot		
Multibran, creamy, instant, dry	¼ cup	8.0
Oat bran	⅓ cup	5.0
Oatmeal, cooked	¾ cup	1.6

Food	Portion	Fiber (g)
Fruit		
Figs, dried	5	8.7
Pear	1 large	6.2
Blackberries	½ cup	4.5
Dates	5	3.2
Orange	1	3.1
Raspberries	½ cup	3.1
Prunes	5	3.0
Apple, with skin	1	3.0
Strawberries	¾ cup	2.9
Apricots, dried	10 halves	2.7
Kiwifruit	1	2.6
Nectarine	1	2.2
Cantaloupe	½ melon	2.0
Raisins	¼ cup	1.9
Banana	1	1.8
Plums	3 small	1.8
Blueberries	½ cup	1.7
Apricots	2	1.5
Grains		
Corn bran, raw	1 oz.	23.0
Wheat bran, toasted	1 oz.	14.1
Rice bran, raw	1 oz.	6.2–9.5
Bulgur, raw	1 oz.	5.2
Barley, raw	1 oz.	4.9
Oat bran, raw	1 oz.	5.0
Wheat flour, whole-grain	1 oz.	3.6
Cornmeal, whole-grain	1 oz.	3.1
Wheat germ	1 oz.	3.0
Oats, rolled, dry	1 oz.	2.9
Millet, hulled, raw	1 oz.	2.4

(continued)

Good Fiber Sources—*Continued*

Food	Portion	Fiber (g)
Legumes		
Baked beans, vegetarian, canned	½ cup	9.8
Kidney beans, cooked	½ cup	9.0
Pinto beans, cooked	½ cup	8.9
Black-eyed peas, cooked	½ cup	8.3
Miso (soybeans)	½ cup	7.5
Chick-peas	½ cup	7.0
Lima beans, cooked	½ cup	6.8
Navy beans, cooked	½ cup	6.8
Lentils, cooked	½ cup	5.2
White beans, cooked	½ cup	5.0
Green peas, cooked	½ cup	2.4
Nuts and Seeds		
Almonds, oil-roasted	¼ cup	4.4
Pistachio nuts	¼ cup	3.5
Mixed nuts, oil-roasted	¼ cup	3.2
Peanuts	¼ cup	3.2
Pecans	¼ cup	2.3
Rice, Pasta, and Tortillas		
Pasta, multigrain		
With quinoa, dry	2 oz.	8.0
With triticale, dry	2 oz.	6.5
With oat bran, dry	2 oz.	6.0
Whole wheat, dry	2 oz.	6.0
Rice		
Wild, cooked	½ cup	5.3
Brown, long-grain, cooked	½ cup	1.7
Tortilla, corn	2 shells	3.1

Food	Portion	Fiber (g)
Snacks		
Crackers		
Stone-ground wheat	1 oz.	3.9
Oat crisps, thin	½ oz.	3.2
Hearty wheat	4	3.0
Rye crisps, thin	½ oz.	3.0
Saltines, whole wheat	5	1.0
Cookies		
Graham crackers, oat bran	1.2 oz.	3.0
Oat plus fruit	2	3.0
Oat bran	2	2.8
Fig bars	2	1.3
Popcorn, gourmet	½ oz.	2.0
Vegetables		
Artichoke, raw	1	6.7
Brussels sprouts, boiled	5	4.5
Mixed, frozen, cooked	½ cup	3.5
Sweet potato, baked	1	3.4
Corn, cooked	1 ear	2.8
Parsley, chopped	1 cup	2.8
Parsnips, cooked	½ cup	2.7
Broccoli, raw, chopped	1 cup	2.5
Potato, with skin	1	2.5
Carrot, raw	1	2.3
Turnip greens, boiled	½ cup	2.2
Spinach, boiled	½ cup	2.1
Asparagus, cut	1 cup	2.0
Cauliflower, cooked	5 florets	2.0
Zucchini, cooked	½ cup	1.8
Cabbage, raw, shredded	1 cup	1.7
Green beans, string, cooked	½ cup	1.6
Tomato, raw	1	1.5

Pectin's Special Talents

Do you have high cholesterol? Diabetes? If you do, your bathroom cabinet probably contains medicines to control these problems. But maybe you should also be looking in the produce compartment of your refrigerator for help. You just might find it—in sweet oranges, crisp apples, crunchy carrots, and tasty nuts and beans.

What's so special about these foods? They all contain a gelatinous fiber called pectin. It's the "glue" that holds together plant cells, and it is found in varying amounts in many fruits and vegetables. Home canners know pectin as a white powder, made from apples or grapefruit skin, that's used to firm up jellies. Producing perfect jam, though, is only a small act in pectin's repertoire of skills.

Researchers have found that pectin is one of the best substances there is for reducing high blood-cholesterol levels.

"As far as I can see, pectin is about the most effective fiber for reducing cholesterol levels," says Sheldon Reiser, Ph.D., director of the Carbohydrate Nutrition Laboratory at the U.S. Department of Agriculture's Human Nutrition Research Center in Beltsville, Maryland. Dr. Reiser recently completed a survey of pectin research.

"There have been a great number of studies, done with very diverse segments of the population, and they have confirmed pectin's role in reducing cholesterol levels," Dr. Reiser says. "The consistency of findings in these studies is very impressive."

Pectin Soaks Up Cholesterol

Studies show that pectin reduces blood levels of a harmful kind of cholesterol, known as LDL (low-density lipoprotein) cholesterol. It does this without also lowering levels of beneficial HDL (high-density lipoprotein) cholesterol. That is important because high levels of HDL cholesterol have been shown to reduce your risk of developing heart disease.

Pectin acts like a sponge in your intestines. It binds components of digestive fluids secreted by the liver and gallbladder. Some of these components, called bile salts, are formed from body stores of cholesterol. Normally, after the bile salts are used to digest food, they are reabsorbed into the body to be recycled. But when pectin combines with bile salts, the intestines can't reabsorb them, and they are excreted. That means the body has to dip into its cholesterol stores to make more bile salts. The more often it must do this, the lower its cholesterol stores, and the healthier your arteries. Studies have shown that pectin can absorb up to four times its weight in cholesterol.

Pectin seems to work best in people whose cholesterol levels are highest, Dr. Reiser says. It's particularly effective in people with a genetic tendency toward high cholesterol levels, reducing their blood cholesterol levels by as much as 19 percent. In people with low to normal cholesterol levels, it has less effect.

How much pectin do you need to consume to see results? That depends, Dr. Reiser says. In most studies, pectin didn't begin to have a significant effect on cholesterol levels until people were getting 6 to 8 grams a day. Most studies found increasingly better results as more pectin was given, although most didn't use more than 15 grams a day.

"The trick is to find the lowest amount that works for you," Dr. Reiser says. You can do that by having a blood cholesterol test taken, then adding, say, 6 grams of pectin a day to your diet for a month, then having another blood test. Then, if you want, try adding another 2 to 4 grams of pectin, and in another month, have a second blood test. There's no good reason to overdo it, Dr. Reiser adds. "Once you get to a certain level of effectiveness, there's no indication that you can improve it by adding even more pectin, although there are enough studies where people have gotten 15 to 20 grams a day of pectin that indicate that it isn't harmful."

Using the chart on page 21 as a guide, you can easily select foods that will help you reach the 6 to 10 grams of pectin each day. You might choose to have an orange with your breakfast, a pear with your lunch, and some brussels sprouts for dinner, for example.

Vitamin C Boosts Effects

A few studies have noted that when extra vitamin C is added to your diet along with pectin, cholesterol levels drop even lower. "The enzyme that starts converting cholesterol to bile acids is activated by vitamin C," Dr. Reiser explains. "With vitamin C you have the enzyme capability in your body to transform cholesterol into bile acids." People deficient in vitamin C produce less bile acid. If you're taking pectin, make sure you also get enough vitamin C. In one study, 15 grams of pectin and 450 milligrams of vitamin C daily were found to be very effective in reducing cholesterol levels.

Conveniently, some pectin-packed fruits and vegetables are also rich in vitamin C.

Diabetics Can Benefit, Too

Pectin also works in ways that can help diabetics keep their blood sugar and insulin levels normal and stable. When it is consumed with a meal or in a glucose-tolerance test, pectin reduces the subsequent rise in blood sugar and in insulin levels.

Pectin may work by slowing the absorption of sugar through

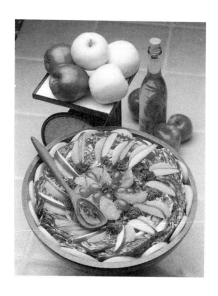

Pectin, the gummy fiber found in the pulp and peel of many fruits and vegetables, helps lower cholesterol, especially when combined with vitamin C. Luckily many foods high in pectin also contain vitamin C, such as oranges and brussels sprouts. Others can be teamed with high-C foods. Here, apples and grapefruit are tossed with cabbage for a healthy salad.

the intestine. "It creates a kind of diffusion barrier on the intestinal lining," Dr. Reiser says. "It creates a thicker membrane barrier through which the glucose has to pass to be absorbed," so sugar is absorbed gradually, through a longer length of intestine.

In studies where pectin was effective in reducing blood sugar and insulin levels, people were getting from 10 to 14 grams with each meal.

Pectin May Help Bowel Disease

Studies done over a number of years have shown that pectin changes the structure of the cells lining the intestine. "In microscopic cross sections of intestinal lining, the villi (tiny, finger-like projections that give the intestinal lining its velvety look) were taller in animals given pectin than in animals on the same diet without pectin," says John Rombeau, M.D., associate professor of surgery at the University of Pennsylvania Medical School. Studies have confirmed that there is more intestinal cell turnover and growth in animals supplemented with pectin.

In trying to see if these findings have any practical application, Dr. Rombeau decided to look at inflammatory bowel disease.

He found that in rats with experimentally induced colitis, those that had pectin added to their diet healed much faster than those fed a fiber-free liquid diet. A study of the pectin-supplemented rats' intestinal cells showed more growth and bigger cells.

During a flare-up of colitis, standard medical treatment is to rest the bowel by stopping food and giving intravenous nourishment, Dr. Rombeau says. "Instead of doing that, we are trying to 'feed' the diseased intestine with a specific fuel that it might utilize."

In the colon, pectin is broken down into what are called short-chain fatty acids. The cells that line the colon can use these fatty acids directly as an energy source. "These fatty acids provide an important source of nourishment for these cells, helping them reproduce, grow, and heal," Dr. Rombeau says.

More research needs to be done before recommendations can be made, Dr. Rombeau notes. But he's hopeful pectin may soon play a role in the treatment of bowel disease. "It's inexpensive, harmless, and may have real potential for patients who need some intestinal healing," he says.

Researchers like Dr. Reiser feel pectin will work best as part of a well-balanced diet that includes plenty of fruits, vegetables, grains, and beans.

"I think there is nothing to lose and everything to gain by eating pectin," Dr. Reiser says. "The foods containing pectin are good for you, and pectin has been shown to be effective. Once people begin to see clinical improvement and feel better, they have the incentive to keep on this kind of dietary regimen."

Sweet Treats Packed with Pectin

One delicious way to get more pectin is to substitute fruits—particularly apples, pears, plums, peaches, and figs—for your usual sugary snacks and desserts. But don't think only in terms of a bowl filled with fruits. Instead, think about fruit with pizzazz. Think watermelon fruit bowl, for example.

Cut the watermelon horizontally, removing one-third.

Where's the Pectin?

It's easy to add more cholesterol-lowering pectin to your diet. By doing so, you'll find yourself eating foods rich in fiber, vitamins, and minerals and low in fat and calories—and that can mean a trimmer you. The table below lists some of the top pectin choices.

Food	Portion	Pectin (g)
Soybeans, mature, dried, cooked	1 cup	2.60
Figs, dried, with skin	5	2.26
Orange	1 medium	2.21
Chestnuts, dried	1 oz.	2.10
Pear	1 medium	1.83
Potato	1 medium	1.79
Sweet potato, boiled, mashed	½ cup	1.31
Brussels sprouts, frozen, boiled	½ cup	1.09
Apple	1 medium	1.08
Papaya	½	1.06
Broccoli spears, frozen, boiled	½ cup	0.97
Banana	1 medium	0.91
Strawberries	1 cup	0.89
Tomato	1 medium	0.86
Hazelnuts, dried, raw	1 oz.	0.85
Lima beans, boiled	½ cup	0.85
Carrot	1	0.78
Pistachios, dried	1 oz.	0.77
Peanuts, dried	1 oz.	0.74
Peach	1 medium	0.70
Peas, boiled	½ cup	0.64
Almonds, dried	1 oz.	0.62
Walnuts, dried	1 oz.	0.57
Green beans, frozen, boiled	½ cup	0.50
Lemon	1	0.46
Summer squash, boiled	½ cup	0.45
Grapefruit	½ medium	0.29
Spinach, raw, chopped	½ cup	0.22

Reserve this top for another use. The watermelon, hollowed out, will be your serving dish for juicy, seasonal fruits. Place balls of cantaloupe, sliced peaches, and whole grapes to create a colorful—and healthful—centerpiece.

Or make a fruit kabob. Alternate wedges of apples, oranges, strawberries, and so forth on skewers and place on a large platter of crushed ice.

And remember when making fresh citrus fruit drinks to toss in parts of the peel. Citrus fruit rind is about 30 pecent pectin—so ''grind the rind'' next time you make a blended drink.

C H A P T E R
T H R E E

Magic Beans and Oat Bran

If you have been told that your cholesterol count is high, do you know what it means? More important, do you know that a simple dietary change can lower it back to normal in a month's time?

Before you can control cholesterol, it's important to understand just what this substance is and how it functions in your body. For starters, cholesterol is not in our bodies merely to cause us trouble. In fact, this fatty, yellow substance—which all humans and animals naturally produce—has a real purpose: It travels in our bloodstream helping to build new cells, produce hormones, and form digestive acids. Every day of your life your body manufactures all the cholesterol you need to get these vital jobs done. What this means is that you don't need to put any more into your body by eating foods that contain cholesterol or boost cholesterol levels.

When you eat a steady diet rich in cholesterol-boosting foods, your body can't use the surplus. So the excess cholesterol begins to build up inside you, forming a waxy plaque which clogs your bloodstream, much like ice jams your household plumbing on a cold day. This buildup causes narrowing of the arteries that lead to your heart. When the arteries become severely narrowed, the blood can't flow through, and you could have a heart attack. If the arteries in your neck that lead to your brain get clogged, you could have a stroke.

According to guidelines set by the National Institutes of Health, you're safe from heart disease if your total cholesterol level is below 200 milligrams of cholesterol per deciliter of blood. (The ideal range is below 180.)

Half of us have blood cholesterol levels over 200, enough to increase our risk for heart disease. Many of us have levels that exceed 250 or 300, putting us at very high risk.

Now for the good news. Fortunately, there is an easy solution to this cholesterol overload—a way to cut cholesterol quickly and safely.

A Diet to Combat High Cholesterol

Based on the latest ground-breaking research by James W. Anderson, M.D., of the University of Kentucky College of Medicine in Lexington and others, the evidence is clear: With the right dietary factors, it's possible to drop your blood cholesterol level 30 points in just 30 days! Granted, some of us may not experience such dramatic results. On the other hand, some of us may fare even better!

Your likelihood of dropping 30 points in 30 days depends on many individual factors, including your current cholesterol level. If your blood cholesterol is under 200 (considered a safe level), your blood cholesterol probably won't drop much further.

The higher your blood cholesterol, however, the more it's likely to drop in response to these dietary changes. In other words, people who have the most to lose—those with the highest cholesterol readings—have the most to gain by following this program.

The cornerstone of the cholesterol cure.   Soluble fiber (so called because it dissolves in water, and prevalent in oat bran and beans) is the star of the exciting cholesterol-lowering research.

In one study, for instance, Dr. Anderson's team studied 20 men, aged 34 to 66, with an average cholesterol level of 260. The men split into two groups. For three weeks, one group added 1½ cups of pinto and navy beans (cooked or in soup) to their daily diets. The other group added a cup of dry oat bran—served as hot cereal and in five muffins—each day.

The men's total cholesterol levels fell 60 points on average.

Fiber affects bad *and* good cholesterol.   The fact is that your body manufactures two kinds of cholesterol. The LDL, or low-density lipoprotein, is the "bad guy" cholesterol known to contribute to heart disease. The HDL—the high-density lipoprotein or "good guy" cholesterol—can reduce your risk of heart disease. All this means that as far as protecting your heart goes, the idea is to have less LDL and more HDL.

And research shows that you can get that healthy equation by eating more soluble fiber. In Dr. Anderson's studies, the LDL—the "bad" cholesterol—dropped a whopping 46 points.

In another study, Dr. Anderson looked at 10 men with cholesterol levels averaging 309 points to see how oat bran and beans work in the long run. Six months into the study, the men's cholesterol levels had dropped an average of 76 points. Their LDL averaged 52 points lower. In men who were monitored for two years, cholesterol and LDL had fallen slightly more. And HDL, the good cholesterol, had gained three points, another indicator of improved protection from heart disease.

Although Dr. Anderson's studies were small and sometimes lacked a control group, he has duplicated his results many times.

How Beans and Bran Cut Cholesterol

Scientists are beginning to understand just how beans and bran may help counteract cholesterol. Apparently, soluble fiber increases the output of digestive fluids that your body normally makes from cholesterol after you finish eating. Your liver then has to make more of these fluids, so it dips into your cholesterol stores to do so. That leaves less cholesterol to circulate in your blood and gum up your arteries.

Other theories hold that soluble fiber surrounds the cholesterol molecules in your digestive tract and carries them out of your body before they can enter your bloodstream.

Better than drugs.   However they work, beans and oats generally do so with fewer side effects than cholesterol-lowering drugs, which can cause liver problems, constipation, and other complications. And lowering cholesterol with soluble fiber is less expensive than drug therapy, according to one study. For someone with a cholesterol level over 265, a year's supply of cholestyramine cost $1,442; colestipol, $879. A year on oat bran, by comparison, cost only $248.

Here's one last reason to supplement your diet with oat bran and beans in preference to drug therapy: They taste good. So, what are you waiting for? Let's get started.

Starting Your Anticholesterol Diet

The basic idea behind an anticholesterol diet is simple: You must add foods that lower your cholesterol level and subtract foods that raise the bad cholesterol.

Then, the key to keeping your cholesterol low is to stick with these dietary changes. You're most likely to stick with changes you make slowly. That's why our four-week or 30-day program works so well. It's just enough time to ease into a healthy transformation. And it's enough time to register a significant (30-point) drop in your cholesterol reading.

Just ask Dr. Anderson's patients. They followed his easy-to-stick-with diet for up to seven years—maintaining low cholesterol all along. Now that's motivation!

Week One

You start your program by concentrating on *adding* foods that help escort the cholesterol out of your body.

Put oat bran on your menu.   Add about ⅓ cup of dry oat bran to your daily diet. You can get that amount in two oat-bran muffins . And try mixing in a bit of oat bran when you make casseroles, croquettes, and burgers.

Drink fluids.   You should drink at least eight glasses of fluid a day. Fiber normally draws water into the intestine—that's how it softens stool. Without enough water, though, fiber sometimes blocks the intestine.

Take a multivitamin/mineral supplement.   There are two reasons for this recommendation. "First, many people may not get enough vitamins and minerals to begin with," says Dr. Anderson. "Second, since we don't know the long-term effects of fiber on vitamin and mineral absorption, we prescribe a supplement as a precaution." Take a daily supplement that delivers 100 percent of the Recommended Dietary Allowance (RDA).

Week Two

If your body has adjusted well to fiber so far, double your intake of soluble fiber. If you like oat bran, aim for ⅔ cup of oat bran per day. To get this amount, you need to eat four oat-bran muffins or two muffins and ⅓ cup of oat-bran cereal each day. (Just make sure you read the cereal labels; some are made with coconut oil, a saturated fat that raises cholesterol.)

Alternate with beans.   One cup of cooked beans contains the same amount of soluble fiber as ⅔ cup of oat bran. Better yet, eat oat bran and beans over the course of the day; two oat-bran muffins for breakfast and a bowl of chili (containing ½ cup of cooked beans) for lunch, for example, will easily fit the bill.

Go for variety.   Legumes are among the most versatile of all foods. Try bean burritos or a hearty bean soup. Toss kidney beans in pasta salad. Puree chick-peas with pickles and low-fat dressing to make a delightful sandwich spread. Or stir-fry vegetables with firm tofu (made from soybeans). Dried or canned beans work just as well. Rinse canned beans before using, however, to reduce added salt. (See chapter 4 for more on the benefits of beans.)

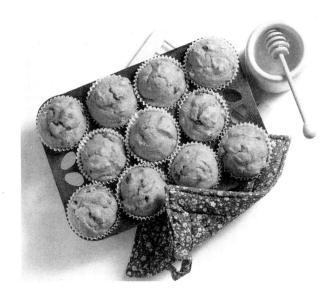

These ordinary oat-bran muffins can offer you extraordinary health benefits you can't get from baked goods made with refined white flour. Consider that one oat-bran muffin packs nearly five times the fiber of a Danish. And if you eat two of these mighty muffins each day, add some beans to your menu, and subtract saturated fat, you can make your cholesterol drop 30 points in 30 days!

Week Three

Continue with the recommendations for Week Two. Then, concentrate on *limiting* foods that boost cholesterol levels in your body. That means you need to trim the saturated fat found in red meat and dairy products from your diet.

An excess of saturated fat, experts say, can drive up the cholesterol level by shutting off the liver's ability to dispose of excess cholesterol. The surplus ends up on our artery walls. And thickened arteries can shut off the blood flow to the heart and brain.

A low-fat diet, on the other hand, can help lower cholesterol and promote overall good health.

Defat your dairy products.   Choose low-fat and nonfat milk over whole milk and select low-fat yogurt and evaporated skim milk instead of heavy cream. Substitute ricotta, part-skim mozzarella, and low-fat cottage cheese for high-fat cheddar or cream cheese.

Choose "lite" spreads and dressings.   On sandwiches, hold the high-fat mayo—light mayonnaise and mustard are better alternatives. On salads, use low-fat dressings. Top your baked potato with a dollop of yogurt and use yogurt instead of mayo to make tuna salad or for substituting for cream in recipes.

Select low-fat snacks.   Munch on air-popped popcorn, pretzels, gingersnaps, and vanilla wafers. Don't forget fruit—a good source of soluble fiber. Prunes, raisins, figs, dates, and apples are good choices.

Limit your egg intake to two yolks a week.   One measly egg yolk contains nearly 300 milligrams of cholesterol. (Egg whites are fine; they don't contain any cholesterol.)

Week Four

Continue with the recommendations for Week Three. Meanwhile, take the final steps to fine-tune your low-fat diet.

Trim the fat off meats and the skin off poultry. When possible, substitute poultry for red meat. Try chili made with chicken and meat loaf made with ground turkey.

Alternate your meat meals with fish.   Choose the darker ocean fish such as mackerel, tuna, or salmon. These dark-meat ocean fish contain omega-3 fatty acids, a type of oil which can reduce blood clots and raise your good cholesterol levels.

Don't fry foods.   Instead, try steaming, baking, broiling, or grilling. If you must fry, grease the pan with a nonstick spray or use nonstick pans.

Eat lean vegetarian dishes when you can.   Try meatless lasagna or pasta with a low-fat sauce as the entrée. Choose red sauces versus white cream sauces.

Limit butter.   Switch to margarine made with pure corn or soybean oil whenever possible. Better yet, choose one of the light whipped tub brands. The softer the margarine, the less hydrogenation it has undergone. Hydrogenation is a chemical process that makes fat saturated, and saturated fat is exactly what you want to avoid.

Substitute olive or canola oils.   These two oils are loaded with monounsaturated fat, one of the good-guy fats shown to reduce cholesterol, and are believed to be healthier for the heart than the polyunsaturated oils like sunflower or other vegetable oils.

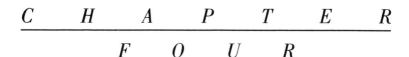

_C H A P T E R_

_F O U R_

Eat Lean with Bean Cuisine

There is growing evidence that fiber-rich food may be one of your best weapons in the war against obesity.

But just how does fiber help you fight excess flab?

"The process begins in the mouth," explains George L. Blackburn, M.D., associate professor of surgery at Harvard Medical School and chief of the Nutrition/Metabolism Laboratory with the Cancer Research Institute at the New England Deaconess Hospital. "High-fiber foods must be chewed—and chewed and chewed. This allows more interaction with your taste buds so you have more sensory satisfaction."

The stomach is the next site where fiber stems the appetite. "The stomach's job is to turn entering solids into a form that's liquid enough to exit," says Dr. Blackburn. "Fibrous foods are an especially tough demolition job. It takes the stomach a long time to produce all the digestive juices, hormones, and enzymes to liquefy fibrous foods. So the stomach feels full longer and sends signals that say, 'Don't send more! I'm not through digesting what you've eaten!'"

In other words, if you bring your fiber count up by increasing whole grains, fruits, and vegetables, you'll be less hungry for fattening foods. And you'll feel satisfied on fewer calories.

That's what University of Alabama researchers found when they allowed people to "pig out" on a low-calorie, plant-based diet. While the selection included chicken, it also offered plenty of fresh fruits, vegetables, whole grains, and beans. Another group had free access to lower-fiber foods such as ham, roast beef, french fries, and desserts. The first group spent more time eating but took in half the calories (1,570 versus 3,000) compared to the second set of diners.

How Fiber Erases Calories

Once eaten, fiber continues combating hunger in the stomach. The type of insoluble fiber in whole wheat products tends to expand by absorbing water, which contribtutes to feelings of fullness. This undigestible roughage won't give up, even in the intestines. Fiber actually erases some of the calories eaten by helping to escort certain dietary fats out of the intestines before they've had a chance to be absorbed. It's been estimated, in fact, that a diet rich in fiber could reduce the number of available calories one eats by about 5 percent, enough to dispose of about 100 extra calories a day.

That most interesting fact was revealed in one study carried out jointly by the U.S. Department of Agriculture and the University of Maryland over a decade ago.

In the study, a dozen adult men were put on a low-fiber diet for 26 days and a high-fiber diet for another 26 days. Although their change in body weight, if any, was not reported, careful analysis revealed that on the high-fiber diet there was a 4.8 percent decrease of digestible calories compared to the low-fiber diet. That's a significant percentage, amounting to 86 fewer calories a day absorbed on a diet consisting of 1,800 calories and 120 fewer calories a day absorbed from a diet of 2,500 calories.

The researchers found that 96.3 percent of the calories consumed in the low-fiber diet were absorbed, and only 91.6 of those in the high-fiber diet actually passed through the intestinal tract and into the system where they could provide energy—and fat power.

Fiber counteracts constipation.   "Insoluble fiber is a bulking agent, which means it prevents constipation," says Dr. Blackburn. "Constipation—and the draggy feeling that comes with it—are common among dieters because they are eating less food. Not only is constipation uncomfortable, but at our weight-loss clinic at the New England Deaconess Hospital we've found that less-constipated dieters have an easier time sticking to a weight-loss regimen."

The best way to beat bingeing.   Fiber can be a boon to dieters in yet another way. In large amounts, soluble fiber—the kind found in oat bran, beans, barley, and some fruits and vegetables such as apples, cabbage, and potatoes—can keep the blood sugar levels steady. That's especially useful for dieters. On a low-fiber diet, your metabolism runs up peaks and down valleys, causing sudden energy losses and jittery feelings that can trigger bingeing. But soluble fiber helps keep your metabolism—and your appetite—on an even keel.

High-fiber foods also tend to lower circulating levels of insulin, a hormone that is believed to stimulate appetite. They probably do that simply by making you need less insulin.

Beans: The Very Best Diet Food

The evidence is clear: People who are actively losing weight should make a special effort to select the highest-fiber foods.

What foods fit that bill? Complex carbohydrates—foods like whole grains, fresh fruits and vegetables, and beans.

Yes, beans. The humble, oft-ignored bean may just be the perfect diet food. Beans are classified as legumes, the dried seeds of pods. A cup of most common varieties weighs in at around 225 to 250 calories. And it's what you get for those calories that makes beans such a lean choice.

After all, it's not just calories that count in a weight-loss program. It's cutting fat, because dietary fat readily adds fat to your frame; and boosting fiber, which fills you up, not out; and focusing on foods that pack maximum nutrition in every calorie.

Beans may be your best bet because they are an excellent source of complex carbohydrates, packed with fiber and containing almost no fat.

Beans are nuggets of nutrition.   With a rich, meaty flavor, beans can easily muscle aside the fat-heavy meat on your plate. And because they contain amino acids (which combine with other amino acids in rice, grains, or pasta to form complete proteins), your body won't miss the meat protein.

Best of all, beans are about as nutrient-dense a food as you're likely to find. They boast healthy doses of anemia-fighting iron, nerve-soothing B vitamins, and bone-building calcium and phosphorus—nutrients that fall short on many dieters' menus. Some varieties also have magnesium, manganese, and potassium.

The bottom line on beans.   According to Sonja L. Connor, R.D., research assistant professor of clinical nutrition at Oregon Health Sciences University, most of us would do well to gradually increase our consumption to three to five cups of legumes a week. To make room, trim your diet of fatty meats and empty-calorie foods. You'll be glad you did. After all, any food with a nutritional profile like this can't help but improve your own profile.

A Buyer's Guide to Beans

You can't get bored with beans: There are so many varieties available, including black beans, navy (or northern) beans, chickpeas, black-eyed peas, split peas, kidney (red) beans, fava beans, pinto beans, lima beans, soybeans, and lentils (which range from brown to green or coral).

Among the most popular dried beans are mung, pinto, kidney, Great Northern, and navy beans. They're good sources of the

B vitamins thiamine and B_6, and they also contain significant amounts of niacin, folate, calcium, iron, magnesium, and potassium.

Best of all, dried beans are a fantastic source of fiber. Consider that a serving of navy beans packs a whopping 9.6 grams of fiber, as much as four slices of whole wheat bread. A half cup of kidney beans provides about 4 grams of fiber—a very respectable amount; the same amount of pinto beans delivers even more.

How to buy beans in bulk.   As far as buying dried beans goes, they are commonly sold in 1-pound packs. If you're buying them from bulk bins, choose whole, unbroken specimens that are uniform in size with clear, bright colors and a nutty aroma. Store them in glass jars in a cool cupboard or the refrigerator. They'll keep for a year. Adding a pinch of rosemary or a bay leaf to the jar will help beans stay fresh.

Canned beans come in handy.   Although canned beans tend to contain slightly less of some nutrients due to the heat processing they undergo, they're still a good food and are convenient when you haven't precooked any dried beans. Be aware, though, that a lot of sodium is added during canning. For best results in terms of both taste and health, place the canned legumes in a strainer and rinse with cool water until it runs clear, about 30 seconds. This will eliminate much of the excess salt. Then use them interchangeably with precooked dried beans in recipes.

Prepping Beans for Easy Digestion

Beans have a bad reputation for producing gas. The problem is they contain certain water-soluble starches that the body cannot break down during digestion. But the key here is ''water-soluble.'' By repeatedly soaking the beans in water (and discarding the runoff), much of the problem can be eliminated. Here's how:

1. Start with a pound (2 cups) of dried beans. Discard any that are broken or discolored. Rinse until the water runs clear.
2. Place the beans in a large soup pot with 6 cups of cold water. Boil for 2 minutes.
3. Drain the water, and replace it with fresh. Let stand overnight or for at least 6 hours.
4. Drain well. Add fresh water. Bring to a boil, then simmer, loosely covered, until the legumes are tender (start checking lentils after 30 minutes; others will take up to 2 hours).

Note: To save time, prep the beans ahead and store for later use. Beans prepared as above can keep for a week in the refrigerator or 6 months in the freezer. (Don't freeze lentils, however; they turn mushy.)

Timetable for Cooking Beans

Beans take time to cook—but the wait is well worth it. When the time is up, you'll have one of nature's best diet aids ready to include in any number of tasty and filling dishes. To prepare your beans, wash them, cover them generously with water, and soak them overnight (lentils and split peas need no soaking). Drain, then place the beans in a saucepan and cover with water. Bring the water to a boil, reduce heat, and simmer until tender.

Type of Bean	Cooking Time
Lentils	45 minutes
Split peas	1 hour
Navy beans	1 ½ hours
Lima beans	1 ½ hours
Kidney beans	1 ½ hours
Black beans	1 ½ hours
Chick-peas	3 hours
Soybeans	3 hours or more

Five Ways to Bean Up Your Diet

You can sneak beans into just about any soup, stew, salad, or stuffing. Here's how:

- Puree cooked legumes in a food processor or blender. Stir in minced garlic, basil, and thyme to taste. Use as a low-fat spread for crusty bread or crisp vegetables.
- Chop cooked beans as a high-fiber, low-fat substitute for the meat in lasagna.
- Add cooked legumes to soups, stews, stir-fries, casseroles, meat loaves, and omelet fillings.
- Substitute cooked beans cup for cup for the bread cubes in poultry stuffing.
- Marinate cooked legumes in herbed vinegar with a splash of olive oil. Toss into vegetable or green salads.

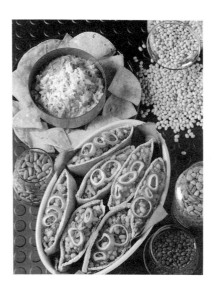

Watching your weight? Try a pita sandwich stuffed with savory chickpeas and onions. Chickpeas and other beans are slow to digest, so you feel full longer. Beans also can fight flab. Studies show that overweight people lost pounds simply by adding fiber to their diets—with no other dietary changes!

Best High-Fiber Breakfasts

Of the three main meals you eat, breakfast is the most important. A hearty breakfast can refuel your energy levels and help you get off on the right foot.

Unfortunately, many people skip breakfast or else grab a jelly doughnut or a sugar-laden Danish on the run. Little wonder that they feel dragged out by midmorning. That sweet dose romances your blood sugar way up—and then drops it, leaving you in a funk of fatigue.

Other people go to the opposite extreme—they stoke up on a big platter of eggs, fried potatoes, and bacon, sausage, or ham. The traditional bacon-and-eggs breakfast can easily pack a gram of fat *in each bite*.

But with whole-grain breads, muffins, cereals, or hotcakes, you can wake up to breakfasts that are hearty and healthy and hit the spot—without hitting you with a bunch of empty calories.

In fact, studies show that when you breakfast on whole grains, you'll probably *lose* weight, since with grains a little goes a long way. With so much fiber, grain products can help reduce your calorie intake because you feel fuller longer.

In one study 14 volunteers started off their morning with a bowl of one of five cereals—ranging from low to high fiber content. After 3½ hours, they were guided to a buffet where they were invited to graze on burgers, peanut butter, pickles, corn chips, and other munchies. Those who ate the highest fiber cereal for breakfast ate about 45 calories less than average at the buffet.

Another study showed that people who started their day with the high-fiber cereal ate fewer calories (an average of about 90 fewer) at lunch. Their calorie consumption—breakfast plus lunch—was also lower.

And that's not all. Soluble fiber—prominent in oat bran—helps keep your blood cholesterol under control. Finally, insoluble fiber—most associated with wheat bran but also found in other whole grains—may help prevent colon cancer, some researchers speculate. Both types of fiber get your day off to an A1 start.

A Guide to Ten Great Grains

Grains are probably the least expensive but richest source of nutritional rejuvenation around.

But just what is a grain? Basically, it's a seed—a seed composed of the *germ* (which allows the seed to germinate), the *endosperm* (the starchy part that nourishes the seedling during its early growth), and the *bran* (the protective outer hull). Whole grains have all three parts and are delicious.

While you're experimenting with eating more grains, you also may want to experiment with different kinds of grains. There's more in the world than just whole wheat, after all. Research shows that other types of grains—such as buckwheat and oats—deserve a place at your breakfast table and at each meal because of some special nutritional characteristics.

The following guide can help you expand your grain repertoire.

Amaranth. This is not yet a household grain, but it could be someday. The "mystical grain of the Aztecs" has high quality, more of the amino acid lysine than any other grain, plus significant amounts of iron and magnesium. Look for it in new health-food products like cereal and pasta.

Barley.   Available as pearl barley (which is white and translucent and has had its outer husk removed) and pot, or Scotch, barley (which has had only a single outer layer removed and must be soaked overnight before cooking). Either makes a delicious pilaf when cooked in broth with mushrooms and onions. Also used to flavor and thicken soups and stews.

Buckwheat groats.   It's grain*like,* but it's not a grain. Strictly speaking, it's a fruit, and that means that unlike wheat and rice, the buckwheat seed has no bran or germ; it's simply a kernel wrapped inside a shell. The kernel, called a groat, is the edible part. Buckwheat groats are usually served as breakfast cereal, in puddings, or as a stuffing for meat or poultry.

More popular, though, is kasha—roasted buckwheat groats. Kasha has a nutlike flavor and is a traditional Eastern European food.

Nutritionally speaking, buckwheat is superb. Its protein efficiency is better than any grain's; buckwheat is especially well endowed with the amino acid lysine, a substance that most of the true grains lack. By combining buckwheat with oats, wheat, or rice, you can create a very high-quality protein source. Buckwheat is also a fair source of B vitamins, especially B_6, and iron.

Bulgur.   A traditional food in the Middle East and Asia, since ancient times bulgur has been prepared by first boiling or roasting the raw wheat grain and then spreading it out to dry in the sun. The hard, dry wheat berries are then rubbed by hand to remove some of the bran, sprinkled with water, and then cracked in a mortar and pestle. Modern milling techniques have refined and streamlined these steps, but they remain basically the same.

The result is a hard, partially dehulled, cracked wheat that swells up during cooking to roughly double its size. Bulgur is amazingly versatile and can be eaten for breakfast as a cereal, used as an extender in meat, poultry, or fish dishes, added to bread dough or pancake batter, and added to soups as a rice or noodle substitute; it can even be eaten plain.

Astoundingly, many of the nutritional benefits of raw wheat are retained during the production of bulgur. The amounts of the B vitamins riboflavin and niacin are nearly equal in wheat and bulgur, as are iron and calcium. It also retains a full 75 percent of its fiber.

Cornmeal.   Available in white, yellow, and blue varieties—the blue is favored in Tex-Mex and American Indian foods—cornmeal can be used to thicken sauces, gravies, and soups. It can also be made into polenta and used in unleavened breads, pones, muffins, griddle cakes, and tortillas.

Millet.   These tiny yellow kernels are probably more familiar to you as birdseed. But it's foolish to say that millet is simply for the birds. As is true of all grains, millet is a good source of the B vitamin thiamine and of the minerals iron and magnesium. And you don't have to peck millet out of a tiny cup. It can be used as a rice substitute, as a hearty breakfast cereal, or as an addition to stews, soups, bread dough, and other baked goods.

Oats.   By now, oats are probably no stranger to you. But they are far more versatile than the main ingredient in oatmeal and muffins. For one thing, oats come in two varieties. Steel-cut oats are made by cutting the groats into pieces with steel rollers. Rolled oats, the more familiar form sold for cooked oatmeal, is steamed and flattened by rollers before being packaged, and yet the result is still nutritious enough to be considered a whole-grain product. The so-called quick-cooking oats are precut, steamed, and flattened even more; and instant rolled oats are quick oats with guar gum added, a substance that thickens them to oatmeal-type consistency in less than a minute. Although the more-processed varieties don't lose many nutrients, they often gain sugar and artificial ingredients, so your best bet is still plain old rolled oats.

As you may recall from chapter 3, eating oat bran is one good way to protect your heart. Studies show that oat bran can lower the levels of LDL cholesterol (low-density lipoprotein cholesterol—the harmful stuff of which hardened arteries are made) in the blood while it raises (or leaves intact) the levels of HDL cholesterol (high-density lipoprotein—the beneficial form of blood lipid).

For this reason, you would be wise to try and work a serving or two of oat bran into your daily menu. Use it to thicken and enrich soups or to extend meat dishes. Also great in stuffings, pilafs, breads, pancakes, and granola.

Quinoa.   This grain was a staple of the ancient Incas, who dubbed it the ''mother grain.'' It contains more protein than any other grain and is higher in unsaturated fats and lower in carbohydrates than most other grains. The tiny bead-shaped grain cooks like rice and expands up to four times its original size. Use it the way you would rice—in main dishes, side dishes, in soups and salads. You can buy it packaged as a grain, ground into flour, and in several forms of pasta.

Rye.   Rye is a nutritious cereal grain, and rolled into a flake it can be added easily to granola-type cereals. Coarsely ground rye meal and finely ground rye flour can be blended with other kinds of flour to produce new tastes in bread and other baked goods.

Light rye is like white flour: It's chemically bleached, has next to no bran, and is a nutritional washout. Pass it by.

Triticale.   This is a hybrid of wheat and rye and contains more protein and less gluten than wheat. It has a nutty-sweet flavor and comes in several forms including whole berry, flakes, and flour. Use it in cereals, casseroles, and pilaf-style dishes.

Fiber-Rich Ways
to Start Your Day

Eating your fair share of fiber does not necessarily mean you have to eat a boring bowl of cereal for breakfast every day. You can vary your morning diet with pancakes, crepes, waffles, and porridge. Substitute buckwheat flour for all or part of the regular unbleached flour in your favorite waffle recipe, for example. Or look for whole-grain waffle and pancake mixes at your health food store.

You can also liven up your cereal with a mix of grains such as rolled oats and wheat germ. And top it off with fresh and dried fruit, for a double dose of fiber.

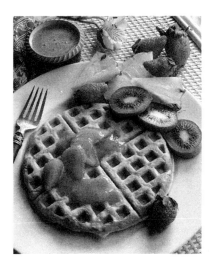

For an eye-opening breakfast, try whole-grain waffles, pancakes, crêpes, or muffins made with not-so-run-of-the-mill grains like barley, bulgur, and cornmeal. The waffles shown here, topped with a tangy berry sauce, owe their tasty goodness to buckwheat and buttermilk.

With a little creativity, even toast can take on a healthy new dimension. Here's French toast with a new American twist: Start with a loaf of oat bread. Slice it, dip it in a seasoned egg-white-and-skim-milk batter. Pan-fry it with nonstick spray. Then top it with your favorite all-fruit conserve. *Voilà:* a low-fat, cholesterol-lowering creation!

C H A P T E R
S I X

Make Room for Rice

Are you watching your weight? How about your cholesterol? Maybe your sodium intake? Are you searching for a food that's filling, satisfying, *and* low in calories? Rice measures up on all counts, and it's high time you recognized this grain for the exciting, healthy food it is.

Besides being light on calories, rice is incredibly low in fat and sodium (as long as you cook it without added fat and salt). It's free of gluten and nonallergenic. Rice is also a source of fiber, thiamine, riboflavin, niacin, and iron (the exact amounts vary according to the type of rice).

Brown rice is the top gun as far as fiber or other nutritional benefits go. It's undergone very little processing, having had only its inedible outer hull removed. Because the brownish bran that gives it its color is intact, there's three times more fiber present than in white rice. Nevertheless, white rice remains an important staple in healthy diets worldwide. This suggests that, even in its refined state, rice is intrinsically good food and should be included as a regular part of your diet.

Name That Rice

There are an estimated 7,000 varieties of rice worldwide. You're not likely to find most of them at your corner market. But don't be surprised to discover some unusual varieties, such as Basmati (from India) or Texmati (an American hybrid)—both slightly nutty in flavor—or arborio (from Italy), cropping up on your supermarket shelves next to brown, white, and wild rice.

Rice is classified by the length of its grains and basically falls into the following three types.

Long grain.   This is by far the most popular rice around. It includes the aromatic varieties, such as Basmati and Texmati.

Rice Bran Rivals Oat Bran

If you are stuck in the oat-bran-for-breakfast rut, here's a great new way to spark your morning meals— reach for the rice bran. If a preliminary study is confirmed, researchers can say that rice bran may rival oat bran in cholesterol-cutting power.

The study, led by Talwinder S. Kahlon, Ph.D., research nutritionist at the U.S. Department of Agriculture Western Regional Research Center in Albany, California, tested high-fiber diets in hamsters. When 10 hamsters spent three weeks on a high-cholesterol diet with 10 percent of dietary fiber from oat bran, their cholesterol, as expected, dropped significantly.

But when fed rice bran (sold in health-food stores and specialty shops), the hamsters' cholesterol dropped as much as it had on the oat bran.

The study hasn't yet been reviewed by other scientists, and rice bran has yet to be tested in humans. But if you'd like to try rice bran, start with this moist muffin. It combines rice bran with the proven cholesterol-cutting power of oats and monounsaturated oil.

(continued)

Rice Bran Rivals Oat Bran—
Continued

Rice Bran Muffins

Muffins

2	cups rice bran	¼	cup water
2	cups quick-cooking oats	1	tablespoon canola oil
2	teaspoons baking soda	3	egg whites
½	teaspoon salt	1	teaspoon vanilla extract
½	cup brown sugar		grated rind of one orange
1	cup nonfat yogurt		
1	cup unsweetened applesauce	1½	cups blueberries

Topping

½	tablespoon granulated sugar	1	teaspoon cinnamon

Muffins: Preheat oven to 400 °F. Line muffin tins with paper liners.

In a large bowl, combine bran, oats, baking soda, salt, and sugar.

In a medium bowl, blend yogurt, applesauce, water, oil, egg whites, and vanilla. Combine liquid ingredients with orange rind and dry ingredients. Mix thoroughly but don't beat.

Stir in blueberries. Fill muffin tins three-quarters full.

Topping: Mix sugar and cinnamon. Sprinkle ¼ teaspoon topping over each filled cup. Bake 20 to 25 minutes.

Makes 18 muffins.

When cooked, the long grains remain separate and fluffy, making them ideal for pilafs, stuffing, rice salad, and casseroles.

Medium grain.   This rice is shorter, plumper, and a bit stickier than long grain when cooked. It can double for long grain in many recipes. Just double-check package instructions before making such a switch because some medium-grain varieties require less water.

Short grain.   This rice is stubby, almost round in shape. When cooked, it's very sticky and somewhat heavy in texture. It's perfect for sushi, croquettes, and stuffed peppers. Arborio is an Italian short-grain rice with an exceptionally creamy texture that's used for risotto.

The Ways of Rice

Forget the adage ''A watched pot never boils.'' When it comes to cooking rice, you're better off keeping a close watch on your boiling pot.

You should also follow this rule of thumb for cooking rice: 1 cup of dry rice requires 2 cups of liquid, but exact measurements and cooking times can vary. (Consult package directions or refer to the table ''Choosing and Using Rice'' on page 48.) Here's one foolproof cooking technique that works for most.

Bring the liquid to a boil, add the rice, and allow it to boil uncovered for 5 minutes. Reduce the heat to a gentle simmer and partially cover the pan (leave the lid just slightly ajar). Cook until all the liquid has been absorbed and the grains are tender. If the rice is not tender, add a bit more liquid and continue cooking. The rice is done when all the water has been absorbed and the grains are tender.

Cooking rice is a cinch.   For more rice-perfect cooking tips, read on.

- Some recipes call for rinsing rice before cooking. Wash-

Choosing and Using Rice

Here's a quick rundown for some of the most common types of rice and the amount of liquid and estimated cooking time required to prepare each type.

Type (1 cup)	Liquid (cups)	Cooking Time (min.)	Characteristics
Arborio	3–4½	25–45	Short-grain white from Italy; use primarily for risotto; remains slightly al dente when cooked.
Aromatic, brown	1¾–2½	30–45	Long grain; high in fiber; has aroma similar to brown rice, nuts, corn, corn bran, or hay; includes the brown hybrids, such as Texmati, Pecan, and Wehani; good for curries, Cajun cuisine.
Aromatic, white	1¼–2	15–20	Long grain; has same aroma as brown; includes true white, Basmati, and U.S. hybrids.
Brown	1¾–3	45–60	Higher in fiber than white; comes in long, medium, and short grains; pleasantly nutty flavor; slightly chewy; beige color; unlimited uses.

ing lessens the nutritional value of the finished product. Most domestic long-grain rice needs no rinsing.

- Get wonderful flavor from any type of rice by cooking it in stock instead of water and by adding minced vegetables and herbs to the liquid. A little lemon juice in the liquid has a slight bleaching effect that whitens white rice as it cooks.
- For best results, don't stir rice as it cooks. That tends to release starch within the grains, causing them to stick together and become gummy.
- For variety, lightly sauté the uncooked rice in just a

Type (1 cup)	Liquid (cups)	Cooking Time (min.)	Characteristics
Converted (parboiled)	2–2½	20–25	Long-grain white; bland flavor; grains stay separate when cooked; has undergone a special pressure and steam treatment prior to milling that preserves vitamins; good for pilafs.
White	1¼–2¼	15–20	Comes in long, medium, and short grains; bland flavor; soft texture; pure white color; unlimited uses.
Wild	2½–4	35–50	Not a true rice; is the seed of an aquatic North American grass; difficult to produce; very expensive; deep brown color, chewy texture; slightly smoky, nutty flavor; often mixed with white or brown rice.

little oil until golden in color. That adds flavor and makes the rice less likely to boil over as it cooks.
- You may also bake rice. Place it in an ovenproof dish. Add boiling liquid and any other ingredients. Cover and bake at 350° to 400°F until tender. Exact time will depend upon the temperature and type of rice used, but baking often takes a little longer than stove-top preparation.
- To save time, especially when making brown rice— which takes twice as long to cook as white—prepare a large potful to last several days.

- Store cooked rice tightly covered in the refrigerator. It will keep for about a week. For longer storage, freeze cooked rice in 1- or 2-cup containers.
- To reheat refrigerated rice, spoon it into a tight-mesh strainer and steam over boiling water until hot.
- An alternate method is to warm rice in the microwave. Place in a glass pie plate and sprinkle with 1 tablespoon of liquid per cup of rice. Cover with vented plastic and microwave on full power until hot (about 1 minute for a cup).
- To reheat frozen rice, let it thaw for a day in the fridge and proceed as above. Or place the frozen rice in a microwave dish and heat on full power for about 2 minutes per cup. Stop often to break up the thawing block with a fork, especially if doing more than 1 cup. That way you can gauge how fast the rice is thawing so you don't overcook or dry out the outer kernels.
- Store all uncooked rice in tightly sealed containers in a cool, dry, semidark place. Tear the instructions from the original box and place in the container for later reference. Because brown rice is more perishable than white, store it in the refrigerator or freezer.

Whether you choose short grain, long grain, or medium grain, white, brown, or wild, rice is an important source of fiber and can make a dazzling centerpiece. Here, the unique combination of fresh green peas and bright red radishes adds eye-popping color and tantalizing texture to plain brown rice.

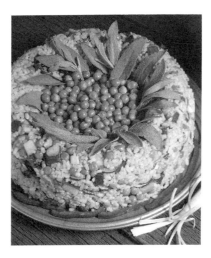

C H A P T E R
S E V E N

Five-Star Recipes

To bulk up your diet with more fiber, you don't have to face a small mountain of bran and tree bark every morning. By now you know that fiber comes in many delicious forms. We're talking about raspberries. Crunchy nuts. Potatoes, blueberries, baked beans, granola . . . the list of good-tasting, good-for-you fiber foods is endless.

The following recipes prove that your familiar fiber-rich foods don't have to bore your taste buds. Here you'll find your fiber favorites prepared in exciting new ways—plus dozens of tantalizing ways to fix the not-so-common forms of fiber as well.

Sample several of these recipes and see for yourself how easily fiber fits into just about any meal—or can even become the starring attraction.

You may even get some ideas for concocting your own high-fiber recipes or embellishing your favorite dishes.

Bon appétit!

Appealing Appetizers

Hors d'oeuvres can play a supporting role by setting the tone for a meal, or they can perform solo at a party. More than just something to nibble on, they can become tiny nuggets of nutrition. Either way, these star appetizers can enhance your healthy lifestyle, providing you bypass the usual, boring hors d'oeuvres—the greasy chips and the dip made from soup mix and fattening sour cream.

Instead, to introduce an elegant dinner, look to Minted Pink Grapefruit Sections, served in a stemmed goblet. Or set the stage

---

Minted Pink Grapefruit Sections

2	large pink grapefruit	1	teaspoon sunflower oil
1	tablespoon shredded fresh mint		mint sprigs (garnish)

Peel grapefruit, removing all of the white membrane. Use a sharp knife to remove sections from membranes, catching any juice in a small bowl.

In a medium bowl, toss grapefruit with mint, oil, and grapefruit juice. Place the sections in small bowls set over crushed ice. Garnish with mint sprigs.

Makes 4 servings.

Variation: Add fresh orange sections to the grapefruit and garnish with thin strips of orange rind.

---

with a stunning arrangement of fruit, which guests dip into a tangy combination of cottage cheese, yogurt, and fruit juice, with just a hint of curry to add interest.

For a little excitement, go Middle Eastern. Tabbouleh-Stuffed Mushrooms make this Lebanese salad stand-up party fare. Try Hummus Tahini, a chick-pea and sesame dip that tastes terrific with pita bread or raw vegetable sticks.

Mexican food buffs will have a fiesta with the savory Mexican Bean Dip—Olé!

Any one of these recipes will enrich any meal that follows with a healthy dose of fiber.

Hummus Tahini

2	tablespoons chopped parsley	½	cup water
2	cloves garlic, minced	2	cups cooked chick-peas
½	cup sesame tahini		dash of cayenne pepper
½	cup lemon juice		parsley sprigs
½	cup olive oil		(garnish)

Place chopped parsley, garlic, tahini, lemon juice, oil, and water in a blender. Process on low speed until smooth.

Add half the chick-peas and process on low speed until smooth. Add remaining chick-peas and continue to process until smooth, stopping to scrape down the sides as necessary.

Place tahini in one or more serving bowls. Sprinkle with a dash of cayenne and garnish with parsley. Refrigerate leftovers, tightly covered.

Makes 3 ½ cups.

Mexican Bean Dip

Chili Seasoning

3 tablespoons ground chili pepper	½ teaspoon cayenne pepper
1½ tablespoons ground cumin	½ teaspoon dried rubbed sage
1 teaspoon dried oregano	½ teaspoon ground allspice

Beans

1 cup cooked red kidney beans	1 clove garlic, minced chopped scallions (garnish)
½ cup yogurt	
½ small onion, coarsely chopped	

Chili seasoning: In a small bowl, combine chili pepper with cumin, oregano, cayenne, sage, and allspice. Use immediately or store in a cool, dry place in a tightly covered small jar.

Beans: Place beans, yogurt, onions, garlic, and chili seasoning in a blender. Process on medium speed until smooth. Pour into a small bowl and garnish with chopped scallions.

Serve with cauliflower and broccoli florets, zucchini sticks, cucumber slices, celery sticks, and Jerusalem artichoke slices, along with other favorite raw vegetables, arranged on a large platter around the dip.

Makes 1½ cups.

Tabbouleh-Stuffed Mushrooms

⅓ cup bulgur
⅓ cup water
3   tablespoons lemon
      juice
20 to 24 large mushrooms
½   cup finely chopped
      tomatoes
⅓   cup minced fresh
      parsley
⅓   cup minced fresh
      spinach

¼   cup minced
      scallions
1   tablespoon minced
      fresh mint
3   tablespoons
      sunflower oil
      cherry tomatoes
      (garnish)
      large mint sprigs
      (garnish)

Place bulgur, water, and lemon juice in a large bowl. Allow bulgur to soak for 20 to 30 minutes, or until it is soft and all liquid has been absorbed.

Remove stems from mushrooms. Place mushroom caps in a large saucepan half filled with boiling water. Return water to a boil, then reduce heat, cover, and simmer 3 to 4 minutes, until mushrooms are firm-tender. Drain and allow to cool.

To make the tabbouleh, add tomatoes, parsley, spinach, scallions, mint, and oil to softened bulgur. Toss until well combined.

Spoon tabbouleh into mushroom caps. If desired, cover with foil and refrigerate before serving. Garnish the serving plate lavishly with cherry tomatoes and mint.

Makes 12 to 16 servings.

Salads for All Seasons

Summer days are salad days. And indeed, a crisp green salad spiked with fresh herbs is a great meal on a hot day. The fiber-rich combination of fresh-from-the-garden fruits and vegetables is almost limitless.

But remember that salads can be adapted to any meal of the day, any season of the year. You can make a colorful and crunchy salad by mixing high-fiber raw veggies with a variety of legumes—or even grains, for that matter.

Try these delicious new ways to make salads exciting—any time of year.

Potato and Raspberry Salad

1	pound small potatoes	1	tablespoon orange juice
1½	cups raspberries	¼	teaspoon Dijon mustard
½	cup snipped chives	⅛	teaspoon grated nutmeg
2	tablespoons canola oil		
1	tablespoon raspberry vinegar		

Steam potatoes for 8 to 10 minutes, or until easily pierced with a fork. Set aside to cool, then cut into bite-size pieces.

In a large bowl, combine potatoes, raspberries, and chives.

In a cup, whisk together oil, vinegar, orange juice, mustard, and nutmeg. Pour over potatoes and toss gently.

Makes 4 servings.

Lentil and Walnut Salad

1 cup lentils
3 cups water
1 carrot
1 tablespoon low-sodium soy sauce
10 sprigs parsley
¼ teaspoon whole cloves
1 clove garlic, peeled
½ cup chopped walnuts
2 tablespoons olive oil
2 tablespoons Sour Yogurt-Cream*

1 tablespoon minced shallots
⅛ teaspoon ground toasted cumin seeds
¼ cup minced fresh parsley
read leaf lettuce
sweet red pepper rings (garnish)
green pepper rings (garnish)

Place lentils, water, carrot, soy sauce, parsley sprigs, cloves, and garlic in a medium saucepan. Bring the water to a boil, reduce heat, cover, and simmer just until tender, 25 to 30 minutes. Drain any liquid and remove garlic, carrot, and as many parsley sprigs and cloves as you can find.

Place walnuts in a small skillet with oil. Sauté just until the walnuts are a light golden brown. Remove from heat.

When the nuts have cooled, add the Sour Yogurt-Cream, shallots, cumin, and minced parsley and stir well until combined.

Gently fold nut and parsley mixture into the lentils.

Arrange the lettuce on a serving plate. Spoon the salad on top of the leaves and garnish with red and green pepper rings. Serve with whole grain crackers and crisp raw vegetables.

Makes 4 servings.

*To make Sour Yogurt-Cream, stir together 1 cup plain yogurt and ½ cup sour cream.

Blueberry-Wheatberry Salad with Honey-Lime Dressing

Dressing

3 tablespoons lime juice
1 tablespoon honey
½ teaspoon dry mustard
¼ teaspoon finely grated lemon or lime rind
⅛ teaspoon paprika
⅛ teaspoon ground coriander
1 egg yolk
½ cup sunflower oil

Salad

1 cup blueberries
1 cup rolled wheatberries
¼ cup finely chopped walnuts
¼ cup minced celery
¼ cup minced red onion
1 tablespoon minced fresh dill
  spinach leaves

Dressing: Place lime juice, honey, mustard, lemon or lime rind, paprika, coriander, and egg yolk in a blender. Process on low speed until combined.

With the blender running, add oil in a slow, steady stream until it's all incorporated. Store in the refrigerator in a tightly covered container.

Makes ½ cup.

Salad: Combine blueberries, wheatberries, walnuts, celery, onions, and dill in a medium bowl. Toss with dressing. Serve on a bed of spinach leaves.

Makes 4 servings.

Soups That Sizzle

Say the word "soup" and the imagination conjures up a steaming bowl that warms both body and soul. Even better than the pleasure it brings, soup is nutritious. In fact, it's hard to find a more pleasant way to use so many forms of fiber.

Forget adding noodles and the same old vegetables to soup. Here are some that use a variety of grains and even fruits to spice up your soup for a meal that stands on its own.

Serve with a hunk of whole-grain bread slathered with fruit butter, and you have a lip-smacking, simmering meal low in fat but loaded with fiber.

Dilled Cabbage Soup

½ medium cabbage, chopped
2 large onions, chopped
1 teaspoon dill seeds
½ teaspoon caraway seeds
1 tablespoon olive oil
4 cloves garlic, minced

1 tablespoon vinegar
3 cups stock
1½ cups tomato juice
1 large potato, diced
2 teaspoons low-sodium soy sauce
¼ cup minced fresh parsley

In a 3-quart saucepan, sauté cabbage, onions, dill, and caraway in the oil, stirring occasionally, until cabbage is translucent and wilted, about 10 minutes.

Add garlic and vinegar and cook for 1 minute. Add stock, tomato juice, potatoes, and soy sauce.

Cover and simmer until potatoes are tender, about 15 to 20 minutes. Add parsley.

Makes 4 servings.

Vegetable Soup with Fennel

3	large ripe tomatoes, peeled, seeded, and coarsely chopped	6	cups water
4	carrots, sliced diagonally	½	cup tomato paste
½	stalk celery, sliced diagonally	1	cup peas (fresh or frozen)

3   large ripe tomatoes, peeled, seeded, and coarsely chopped
4   carrots, sliced diagonally
½   stalk celery, sliced diagonally
1   medium sweet Spanish onion, chopped
1   small fennel bulb, chopped
1   cup corn kernels
⅓   cup barley
6   cloves garlic, thinly sliced
3   tablespoons minced fresh parsley

6   cups water
½   cup tomato paste
1   cup peas (fresh or frozen)
1   cup packed spinach leaves, thinly sliced
1   tablespoon minced fresh dill
2   teaspoons fresh tarragon or ½ teaspoon dried tarragon
2   tablespoons low-sodium soy sauce
    fennel sprigs (garnish)

Place tomatoes, carrots, celery, onions, chopped fennel, corn, barley, garlic, parsley, and water in a kettle or stockpot. Bring to a boil, then reduce heat, cover, and simmer for 1¼ hours.

Add tomato paste. If using fresh peas, add them now and cook 10 minutes. If using frozen peas, add them during the final 5 minutes of cooking. Add spinach, dill, and tarragon and cook 5 minutes longer. Stir in the soy sauce.

Serve hot, garnished with fennel.

Makes 10 servings.

Apple-Barley Soup

2 large onions, thinly sliced	¼ teaspoon dried marjoram
2 tablespoons canola oil	1 bay leaf
3½ cups stock	2 cups chopped apples
1½ cups apple juice	¼ cup minced fresh parsley
⅓ cup pearl barley	1 tablespoon lemon juice
2 large carrots, diced	
¾ teaspoon dried thyme	

In a 3-quart saucepan over medium heat, cook onions in the oil, stirring constantly, for 5 minutes. Reduce heat to medium-low, cover, and cook, stirring frequently, for 20 to 25 minutes, or until onions are golden brown and very soft.

Add stock, apple juice, barley, carrots, thyme, marjoram, and bay leaf. Cover and cook for 1 hour, or until barley is tender.

Add apples, parsley, and lemon juice. Cook for 5 minutes, or until the apples are tender. Discard the bay leaf.

Makes 4 servings.

Loaves You'll Love

If there is one aroma that's most likely to prompt a sense of well-being, it's the heavenly smell of bread in the oven.

But the real treat found in freshly baked bread isn't the smell, it's the taste and the wonderful goodness you know is baked in.

Here are three tasty whole-grain loaves that we've spruced up with crunchy nuts, spiked with herbs, or sweetened with fruits. We've also included an easy-to-bake whole wheat bread that requires no hand kneading and can be whipped up in an hour for a wholesome, loving treat for family and friends.

Banana-Pecan Bread

2 ½	cups whole wheat flour	2 ½	teaspoons baking powder
1	cup unbleached flour	1	cup butter
¼	cup brown-rice flour	1	cup honey
½	cup bran	3	cups mashed very ripe bananas
4	teaspoons ground cinnamon	4	eggs, lightly beaten
		½	cup yogurt
		1	cup chopped pecans

In a large bowl, combine whole wheat flour, unbleached flour, and brown-rice flour. Add bran, cinnamon, and baking powder.

Melt butter in a small saucepan. Remove from heat and stir in honey.

Add butter mixture, bananas, eggs, yogurt, and pecans to dry ingredients and stir just until combined.

Divide batter between two lightly oiled 9 × 5-inch loaf pans. Bake in a preheated 350°F oven for 1 hour, or until a cake tester or knife inserted in the center comes out clean.

Makes 2 loaves.

Easy-Bake Whole Wheat Bread

¼ cup plus ½ tablespoon honey	1 teaspoon salt (optional)
¼ cup warm water	2½ cups hot water
1 package dry yeast	⅓ cup oil
6 to 7 cups whole wheat flour	

Dissolve ½ tablespoon honey in warm water and sprinkle yeast on top. Do not stir. Set aside to proof.

In a large mixing bowl, combine 4 cups flour with salt (if used), hot water, remaining honey, and oil. With an electric mixer, blend on low speed until thoroughly mixed. Add yeast mixture.

Add remaining flour 1 cup at a time, blending after each addition, until dough is consistency of cookie dough. Knead for 10 minutes on low speed.

Grease two large bread pans with solid shortening. Oil hands and mold dough into two loaves. (Lightly oil countertop so dough doesn't stick.) Place dough in pans, cover, and let rise in a warm place until increased in bulk by one-third.

Bake in a preheated 350°F oven for 40 to 45 minutes, or until loaves sound hollow when tapped. Remove from pans and cool on wire racks.

Makes 2 large loaves.

Orange Spice Bread

½	cup butter, melted	⅓	cup unbleached flour
½	cup honey		
½	cup orange juice	2	teaspoons baking powder
½	cup skim milk		
2	eggs	¼	teaspoons ground allspice
¼	teaspoon almond extract		
1½	teaspoons grated orange rind	¼	teaspoon ground cardamom
2	cups whole wheat pastry flour	⅛	teaspoon freshly grated nutmeg

In a large bowl, combine butter, honey, and orange juice. Stir in milk, then beat in eggs until well combined. Add almond extract and orange rind.

In a medium bowl, combine whole wheat flour, unbleached flour, baking powder, allspice, cardamom, and nutmeg. Stir dry ingredients into orange-juice mixture just until combined.

Pour batter into a lightly oiled 8½ × 4½-inch loaf pan. Bake in a preheated 350°F oven for 55 to 60 minutes, until a cake tester or knife inserted in the center comes out clean. Cool on a wire rack.

Makes 1 loaf.

Pesto Party Bread Ring

Pesto Sauce:

⅓ cup virgin olive oil
⅓ cup sunflower oil
⅔ cup unsalted pistachios
2 cloves garlic
¾ cup freshly grated Parmesan cheese

2 cups tightly packed fresh basil
1 cup tightly packed watercress leaves

Bread:

2 tablespoons active dry yeast
½ cup lukewarm water
1 tablespoon light unsulfured molasses
1 tablespoon low-sodium soy sauce

2½ cups buttermilk
½ cup olive oil
1 cup wheat germ
2 cups unbleached flour
5½ to 6 cups whole wheat flour
1 cup pesto sauce

Pesto sauce: Place olive oil, sunflower oil, pistachios, and garlic (pushed through a garlic press) in a blender or food processor. Process on medium speed until mixture is combined but pistachios are just coarsely chopped.

Add cheese and process on medium speed until combined.

Add basil and watercress and process again, stopping to scrape down the sides as necessary, until mixture is nearly smooth. Do not overprocess.

Makes 1½ cups.

Bread: Mix yeast, water, molasses, and soy sauce in a large bowl. Set aside.

Heat buttermilk and oil in a small saucepan until lukewarm.

(continued)

Pesto Party Bread Ring—Continued

When yeast mixture is foamy, stir in buttermilk mixture, wheat germ, and unbleached flour. Beat by hand or with an electric mixer for about 5 minutes.

Stir in enough whole wheat flour to form a kneadable dough. Turn out onto a lightly floured surface and knead until smooth, about 3 minutes.

Break off pieces of dough about half the size of a golf ball. Coat each with some of the pesto sauce. Layer the balls evenly in a buttered Bundt pan or tube pan.

Cover pan with a cloth and allow dough to rise in a warm place until nearly doubled in bulk.

Bake in a preheated 350°F oven for 45 minutes, or until golden brown.

Makes 18 servings.

Hearty Fiber Feasts

Just about any kind of meat, fish, poultry, or vegetable can become a hearty, high-fiber meal with a little creative cookery. Try these change-of-pace main dishes to please your palate:

Chinese Vegetable Pasta

1	tablespoon canola oil	1	clove garlic, thinly sliced
1	large onion, thinly sliced	2	tablespoons low-sodium soy sauce
2	carrots, julienned	1	tablespoon vinegar
1	sweet red pepper, julienned	2	cups cooked vermicelli
1	cup broccoli florets		

In a large nonstick frying pan or wok, heat oil. Add onions and stir-fry for 2 minutes.

Add carrots, peppers, broccoli, and garlic. Stir-fry for 2 minutes.

In a small bowl, stir together soy sauce and vinegar. Pour over vegetables. Add vermicelli and toss well to combine.

Makes 4 servings.

Broccoli and Tofu Stir-Fry

2 large stalks broccoli	1 pound tofu, cubed
3 tablespoons corn oil	dash of cayenne
2 medium onions,	pepper
cut into thin	2 to 3 tablespoons
strips	low-sodium soy
3 to 5 cloves garlic,	sauce
thinly sliced	3 cups hot cooked
1 teaspoon peeled	brown rice
minced gingerroot	

Cut broccoli stalks from florets, then peel stalks and slice thinly on the diagonal. Coarsely chop florets and set aside separately.

Heat oil in a wok or large skillet over medium to medium-high heat until it is hot but not smoking. Stir in onions and broccoli stalks. Cook, stirring constantly, until onions are translucent. Add a few drops of water, as needed, to prevent sticking.

Stir in garlic and ginger, stir a minute or so, then add broccoli florets. Stir until they become a dark green.

Add tofu, cayenne, and soy sauce. Stir, then cover the pan so the vegetables and tofu can steam.

Remove from heat when the vegetables are just crisp-tender. Serve over hot rice.

Makes 4 servings.

Fruit-Topped Perch Fillets

1	cup apple juice		dash of freshly
2	shallots, minced		grated nutmeg
1	apple, thinly sliced	3	cups hot cooked
1½	pounds perch		brown rice
	fillets, with skin	1	tablespoon
1	cup red seedless		arrowroot
	grapes		minced fresh mint
2	oranges, peeled and		(garnish)
	sectioned		
1	banana, sliced		
	diagonally		

Place ¾ cup apple juice, shallots, and apples in a large skillet. Bring to a boil, then reduce heat and simmer about 5 minutes, uncovered.

Add perch in one layer, if possible, over apples. Cover and slowly simmer about 5 minutes.

Top fish with grapes, orange sections, and banana slices. Top with a dusting of nutmeg. Cover pan and cook until fruit is heated through.

Remove fish and fruit carefully from skillet with a spatula and arrange over cooked brown rice. Keep warm.

Mix together remaining ¼ cup of apple juice and arrowroot. Add the juices in the pan and cook over medium heat until slightly thickened. Pour sauce over fruit and fish and serve.

Makes 4 servings.

Chicken Véronique

1	chicken breast, halved, boned, and skinned	⅔	cup apple juice
1	tablespoon safflower oil	2	teaspoons arrowroot
1	tablespoon butter	1	cup seedless red grapes
1	small red onion, chopped	2	tablespoons minced fresh parsley
1	tart red apple, cubed		dash of ground nutmeg
		2	cups hot cooked brown rice

Cut chicken crosswise into ½-inch strips. Place oil in a large skillet, and when pan is warm, add butter. When butter has melted, place chicken strips in pan.

Cook over medium heat until chicken is opaque throughout. Remove from pan with a slotted spoon so the oil and juices remain in pan.

Add onions and apple cubes to the pan. Stir over medium heat until onions are translucent. Add apple juice and simmer until onions are tender, about 10 minutes.

Add arrowroot and stir over low heat until sauce has thickened slightly. Stir in grapes and chicken and heat through.

Stir in parsley and nutmeg, then serve over hot rice.

Makes 4 servings.

Baked Meat Loaf with Pimiento Topping

¾	cup cooked chick-peas	3	tablespoons tomato paste
¼	cup raw sunflower seeds	1	tablespoon low-sodium soy sauce
1	carrot, shredded	8	strips pimiento*
4	scallions, chopped	3	tablespoons water
2	eggs, beaten		parsley sprigs (garnish)
1	pound lean ground beef		
½	cup soft whole wheat bread crumbs		

In a blender, food processor, or food mill, grind chick-peas into meal. (In the blender use short bursts at high speed; in the processor, use the steel blade.) Repeat with sunflower seeds.

Mix chick-pea and sunflower-seed meal with carrots, scallions, eggs, beef, bread crumbs, 2 tablespoons tomato paste, and soy sauce. Pack into a 9 × 5-inch loaf pan.

Decorate top of meat loaf with strips of pimiento. In a small bowl, mix together 1 tablespoon of tomato paste and water. Spoon over top of meatloaf.

Cover pan loosely with foil. Bake in a preheated 350°F oven for 1 hour, removing foil after 30 minutes. Garnish with parsley and serve.

Makes 8 servings.

*Note: To prepare pimiento, place a sweet red pepper under a broiler until the skin is bubbled and charred and the pepper is soft. Wrap in a damp towel for 10 minutes, remove charred skin, and cut pepper into strips.

Desserts without Guilt

Children often prefer dessert over any other part of a meal—and it's a preference many of us never outgrow. Instead of feeling guilty, simply make desserts measure up to your nutritional standards. Prepared wisely, this course can complete the day's balance of essential nutrients and provide one last serving of fiber to round out your daily diet.

Cherry-Maple Crunch

3 cups pitted sour cherries	½ cup rolled oats
1 teaspoon cornstarch	2 tablespoons canola oil
⅓ cup maple syrup	

Coat a 9-inch pie plate with nonstick spray. Add cherries.

In a cup, dissolve cornstarch in maple syrup. Pour over cherries.

In a small bowl, combine oats and oil. Sprinkle over cherries.

Bake at 350°F for about 40 minutes or until lightly browned on top.

Makes 6 servings.

Classic Carrot Cake

Cake

1½	cups whole wheat flour	¼	teaspoon ground allspice
1½	cups unbleached flour	1	cup canola oil
2	teaspoons baking powder	¾	cup egg substitute
½	teaspoon baking soda	¾	cup honey, warmed
1½	teaspoons ground cinnamon	2	cups finely shredded carrots
¼	teaspoon ground mace	1	cup raisins
		½	cup chopped pecans
		1	teaspoon vanilla extract

Frosting

8	ounces Neufchâtel cheese, softened	1	teaspoon vanilla extract
⅓	cup honey, warmed		

Cake: Sift whole wheat flour, unbleached flour, baking powder, baking soda, cinnamon, mace, and allspice into a large bowl.

In a medium bowl, beat oil, egg substitute, and honey until blended. Stir in carrots, raisins, pecans, and vanilla.

Stir liquid ingredients into flour mixture, 1 cup at a time, blending well after each addition.

Coat a 9 × 13-inch baking dish with nonstick spray. Add the batter. Bake at 350°F for 40 to 50 minutes, or until a toothpick inserted in the center comes out clean. Cool on a wire rack before frosting.

Frosting: In a medium bowl, cream together the Neufchâtel, honey, and vanilla until smooth, about 5 minutes.

Makes 20 servings.

Apple Tart

Crust

2	cups rolled oats	1	tablespoon ground cinnamon
¼	cup apple juice concentrate		

Filling

3	large apples, thickly sliced	1	envelope unflavored gelatin
½	cup apple juice concentrate	2	tablespoons honey
½	teaspoon almond extract	2	cups nonfat yogurt
½	teaspoon ground cinnamon	1	cup halved grapes

Crust: In a medium bowl, combine oats, apple juice concentrate, and cinnamon. Press into a 9-inch pie plate. Bake at 350°F for 5 minutes.

Filling: In a 3-quart saucepan, combine apples, ¼ cup of apple juice concentrate, almond extract, and cinnamon. Simmer just until apples are tender, about 10 minutes. Drain and let cool.

In a 1-quart saucepan, place remaining ¼ cup apple juice concentrate. Sprinkle with gelatin and let stand 5 minutes, or until the gelatin is softened. Cook over low heat until gelatin dissolves. Remove from heat and stir in honey.

In a small bowl, whisk yogurt until smooth. Add to gelatin mixture. Pour into crust and refrigerate for 1 hour.

Place apples and grapes over filling in a decorative pattern.

Makes 8 servings.

Heart-Healthy Piecrust

If you love yummy quiches and savory pies but don't want to load up on the saturated fat most pastry crusts supply, you'll be delighted to try this whole wheat version. Olive oil lends some valuable monounsaturated oil to the crust. If you're making a crust for dessert, replace the olive oil with canola oil, another monounsaturate but without the bite.

This recipe makes a standard 9-inch single-crust shell.

Whole-Wheat Pie Shell

2	cups whole-wheat pastry flour	¼	cup ice water
⅓	cup olive or canola oil		

Place flour in a medium bowl and drizzle with oil. Use a pastry blender to evenly distribute oil and produce a mixture that's the consistency of coarse cornmeal.

Sprinkle flour with water, 1 tablespoon at a time, and continue mixing until you can gather dough into a ball.

Roll dough into an 11-inch circle on a pastry cloth. Patch any cracks that may form, but otherwise try not to handle dough more than necessary. Transfer dough to a 9-inch glass pie plate. Trim dough, leaving a 1-inch overhang. Crimp overhanging dough into a decorative edge.

Chill crust for 20 minutes. Fill and bake according to your pie or quiche recipe. For an unfilled crust, prick the shell all over with a fork. Bake it at 350°F for 18 minutes. Let cool before filling.

Makes 1 crust.

Fiber comes in many scrumptious forms, so you can include some in every meal—even dessert. Apples contain both soluble and insoluble fiber. If you make your apple pie with a whole wheat crust, you get another yummy helping of fiber. So dig in and enjoy!

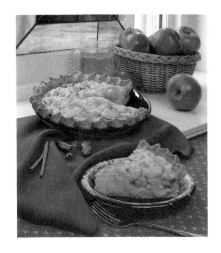

Fiber Meal Plans at Your Fingertips

Throughout this book, we've been telling you that fiber is one of the healing superfoods when it comes to defending you against a variety of diseases such as intestinal and heart disease and obesity. A fiber-rich diet can even protect you against cancer.

In fact, when scientists compare populations that eat fiber-rich diets with those that don't, they find that the high-fiber eaters get less of this deadly disease. That's part of the reason why the National Cancer Institute (NCI) recommends upping fiber intake to 20 to 30 grams a day.

As you may recall from previous chapters, one key to better health seems to be insoluble fiber. The indigestible stalks and peels of fruits and vegetables and husks of whole grains are all examples of insoluble fiber. This roughage bulks up stool and speeds it through the colon. That's why experts theorize that cancer-causing agents are swept quickly away with the stool. And it's also this bulking action of insoluble fiber that may help relieve constipation, hemorrhoids, diverticular disease, and obesity.

You may also recall that when it comes to lowering cholesterol, soluble fiber is the hero. The balance in most fiber foods
tips toward insoluble fiber, but a few (like oat bran and beans)
have an equal amount of soluble fiber. Studies show that some
people can drop high cholesterol levels by eating soluble-fiber-rich
foods while also decreasing total calories.

All this impressive information may have you convinced that
fiber should be an integral part of your diet. But to actually fiber
up your diet is going to take a little effort.

How to Create
a High-Fiber Lifestyle

The fact of the matter is, unless you're sitting under the apple
tree, fiber isn't likely to simply drop into your lap. The typical
American diet provides an average of 11.1 grams per day, not nearly
enough to reap fiber's crop of health-promoting benefits.

With a little know-how, however, it really isn't all that dif-
ficult to get enough fiber. A cup of 100 percent bran cereal, one
apple, one potato with skin, a nectarine, half a cup of split peas,
and half a cup of cooked spinach a day supply about 37 grams—
which is well over the amount of daily dietary fiber recommended
for optimum health.

A fiber formula you can live with.   To help you reach
the recommended fiber intake quota of between 25 and 30 grams
a day, you might want to figure your fiber intake according to your
calorie intake. One formula to follow is to count on 10 to 13 grams
of fiber per 1,000 calories.

Don't go overboard.   The NCI recommends limiting
your intake to 35 grams of fiber a day. Too much fiber may interfere with nutrient absorption and cause intestinal upset.

Double your fiber intake—gradually.   Generally, your
goal is to double your fiber intake. But don't bulk up all at once—
that could cause you intestinal distress followed by a hasty retreat
to low-fiber habits.

It's not a good idea, for example, to wake up tomorrow and

pour bran meal into your breakfast bowl, eat a heaping dish of barley with mushrooms for lunch, and chow down on a big plate of baked beans with broccoli for dinner, plus a couple of apples for snacks. The result of a sudden fiber increase is a day or two of stomach upset, gas, and diarrhea.

"Instead, gradually increase your fiber to give your gut time to get used to it," says George L. Blackburn, M.D., associate professor of surgery at Harvard Medical School and chief of the Nutrition/Metabolism Laboratory with the Cancer Research Institute at the New England Deaconess Hospital. It will take a while for the helpful bacteria that live in your intestine to learn how to break down whole wheat, for example. The products of bacterial fermentation build up, causing bloating and gas. So prepare a sensible plan for adding fiber to your meals.

Allow at least three months to reach your goal. "Most people who want to optimize the amount of fiber they eat should take three to nine months to reach their goal," says Dr. Blackburn. (If you have irritable bowel syndrome, you'll need to stretch that even longer, under medical guidance. It could take two years.)

What to do about gas. If you notice that certain vegetables give you gas—broccoli and cabbage are notorious offenders—eat them cooked instead of raw. Cooking alters fiber's form, but does not significantly decrease the fiber content. Chew slowly and thoroughly to reduce digestive distress.

Go for variety. Don't make the mistake of overindulging in one kind of fiber or another.

What would a day of optimum fiber look like? The table beginning on page 80 illustrates 5 days' worth of delicious food combos that will give you all the fiber you'll need in a day.

The tables and recipes throughout this book can help you choose a good mix of soluble and insoluble fiber foods. As mentioned before, you need both types of fiber for optimum health. Wheat bran, for example, relieves constipation, but it's a matter of some controversy as to whether it can lower cholesterol levels. On the other hand, oat and corn bran can lower blood cholesterol levels. So can pectin, one of the forms of fiber found in pears,

Your Five-Day Fiber-Up Plan

Most experts recommend that an optimal diet should include about 30 grams of fiber a day. As you can see from the following sample meals, this quota is easier to reach than you may think. Keep in mind, however, that these meal plans represent *optimal* fiber intake, and you need to slowly work up to that amount over a period of weeks to allow your system to adjust to your new diet.

Day/Meal	Fiber (g)
Monday	
Breakfast	
1 bowl hot multigrain premium cereal	6.0
with ¼ cup blueberries	0.9
Lunch	
Fruit salad:	
¼ cup raspberries	1.5
¼ cup strawberries	1.0
mixed cantaloupe, honeydew, and watermelon	
balls (equal to ½ cantaloupe)	2.0
½ kiwifruit	1.3
½ cup blueberries	0.9
1 oz. little oat-bran macaroni	3.0
4 oat-bran graham crackers	1.7
Dinner	
2 oz. quinoa multigrain noodles	8.0
with 1 cup asparagus in sesame dressing	2.0
Total	**28.3**
Tuesday	
Breakfast	
2 whole-wheat pancakes	3.6
with ¼ cup raspberries	1.5
Lunch	
Multibean salad:	
¼ cup each of kidney beans	4.5

Day/Meal	Fiber (g)
white beans	2.5
green beans	0.8
1 slice crusty whole-wheat bread	2.3
2 fig bars	1.3
Dinner	
3 brussels sprouts	2.7
½ cup green peas	2.4
½ cup broccoli	1.3
½ cup asparagus tips	1.0
½ cup zucchini	1.8
1 oz. pasta	3.0
Total	**28.7**
Wednesday	
Breakfast	
¼ cantaloupe	1.0
1 bran muffin	2.5
Lunch	
Bowl of chili containing ½ cup kidney beans	4.5
1 oz. stone-ground wheat crackers	3.9
¼ cup raisins	1.9
Dinner	
Tabbouleh	9.5
Hummus containing ¼ cup of chick-peas	3.5
Whole-wheat pita	2.8
Total	**29.6**

(continued)

Your Five-Day Fiber-Up Plan—*Continued*

Day/Meal	Fiber (g)
Thursday	
Breakfast	
2 slices cracked wheat bread French toast	2.6
with ½ pear and cinnamon	3.1
Lunch	
Artichoke	6.7
½ cup wild-rice salad	5.3
with 1 chopped date	0.6
⅛ cup slivered almonds	2.2
½ apple	1.5
Dinner	
Bean tostada:	
¼ cup pinto beans	4.5
1 corn tortilla	1.5
½ cup Mexican brown rice	1.7
Total	29.7

bananas, apples, tomatoes, carrots, and other produce. But neither oat bran nor pectin can relieve constipation.

All this means that you hedge your bets for optimum health when you choose a variety of fiber foods.

Consult your doctor.   If you have kidney disease, diabetes, a bowel disorder, or other serious health problems, get a doctor's go-ahead before increasing your fiber intake. Fiber can produce inflammation or abdominal distress in people whose systems are not equipped to handle it.

Day/Meal	Fiber (g)
Friday	
Breakfast	
1 cup oatmeal-flake cold cereal	6.0
with ½ nectarine, sliced	1.1
Lunch	
Spinach, apple, and cauliflower salad in vinaigrette dressing	5.5
Cup of tomato/barley soup	5.6
4 dried apricot halves	1.1
3 prunes	1.8
Dinner	
Falafel patty containing ¼ cup chick-peas with tomato	3.5
on whole-wheat English muffin	1.5
Corn on the cob	2.8
Total	**28.9**

A Dozen Easy Ways to Fiber Up

Once you become familiar with fiber values (see ''Good Fiber Sources'' on page 12), you'll discover that the best way to boost your intake is to go for the core foods, the heavy hitters in the fiber arena.

Here is a review of the many ways you can boost your fiber intake—and your health—each and every day.

1. Ban the bun for breakfast.   Instead, choose cereals, muffins, waffles, and breads made with whole grains. Wheat-bran cereal is very high in insoluble fiber, while oat bran offers a 50-50 mix of insoluble and soluble. (Oat bran has about three times as much fiber by weight as rolled oats.) But any whole grain can be counted on to make a satisfying, high-fiber breakfast.

2. Mix and match your grains.   Sprinkle a second, crunchier cereal over your bowl of flakes. Stir oat bran into whole-grain pancake batter to add extra soluble fiber. Dried fruits and all-fruit jam provide soluble fiber as well.

3. Invite a legume to lunch.   Kidney beans, lentils, chickpeas, dried beans—are all legumes that are excellent sources of fiber, both soluble and insoluble, and come in enough varieties to keep your palate interested. By the simple act of adding ¼ cup of lima beans to your serving of soup, salad, or casserole, you've upped the insoluble fiber 5.6 grams and the soluble 0.9 grams, for a total boost of 6.5 grams. Substitute beans for some or all of the meat in casseroles. Make tostadas with beans instead of beef.

4. Choose your salad fixings with care.   By supplementing the lettuce and tomatoes in your salad with ¼ cup of raw broccoli and one medium carrot, you add 2.2 grams of insoluble plus 1.5 of soluble fiber—3.7 grams total fiber. And counting a

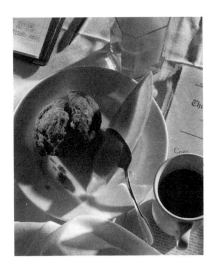

These three meals provide all the fiber you need in a day. **For breakfast:** ¼ *cantaloupe (1.0 gram of fiber) and 1 bran muffin (2.5g).*

half cup of chick-peas, you'll come away from the table 10.2 grams richer!

5. Eat your fruit the way nature grew it.   Choose an apple over applesauce, a whole orange instead of juice. That way you'll get both kinds of fiber, plus all the built-in nutrients. Top-

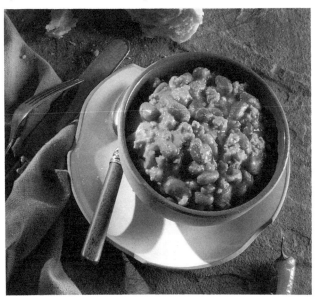

For lunch: *chili containing ½ cup kidney beans (4.5g); 1 oz. stone-ground wheat crackers (3.9g), with ¼ cup raisins (1.9g).* For dinner: *tabbouleh (9.5g), hummus containing ¼ cup chick-peas (3.5g), whole wheat pita pocket (2.8g). Your grand fiber total? 29.6 grams. (The recommended daily fiber amount is 20 to 30 grams.)*

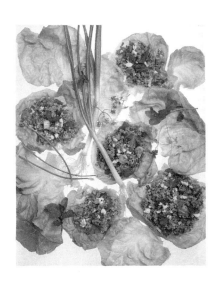

How to Go with the Grain

As you learned in chapter 5, whole grains are one of the best ways to swallow fiber, protein, and a host of vitamins. But cooking whole grains can take a lot of time. If the time crunch sometimes gets in the way of your grain munch, try these super-fast ways to harvest the benefits of whole grains.

- Stock up on whole-grain breads. Try whole wheat pita bread, rich in B vitamins and minerals. Keep pita pockets in the freezer. When you need one, pull it out and toast and stuff the pocket with anything: tuna, cheese, chick-peas, tomatoes, lettuce, bean sprouts.
- Grains make great snacks. Have you tried crunchy rice cakes made of puffed brown rice? They taste like popcorn and make a great base for grilled cheese or spreads. They keep well, too. No need to freeze—seal tightly and store in a dry place.
- Sample sprouted grain bread. Sprouts are super-high in in nutrients, and this kind of bread is

ranking fruits, fiber-wise, are dried prunes, pears, nectarines, and blackberries.

6. Leave the skins on.   Keep fiber-rich peels on apples when you bake them and leave the peels on potatoes when making potato salads.

7. Make desserts a high-fiber affair.   Enjoy an apple tart or fig bar made with whole-wheat flour.

8. Snack sensibly.   Munch on air-popped popcorn, dried fruit, or a whole-wheat pita pocket warmed in the toaster oven.

baked at low temperatures to conserve vitamins.
It also freezes well.

- Try a pasta of a different color. *Udon,* an oriental pasta, is flat, light tan, and made of 100 percent whole wheat. *Soba* is light brown and made of rutin-rich buckwheat. The dark brown *ramen* noodles sold in health food stores are usually composed of whole-wheat flour, buckwheat flour, and sea salt. There's also *superoni,* a soy-fortified American pasta; brown whole-wheat spaghetti; green spinach noodles; and even golden-colored corn spaghetti. All are quick and easy. Experiment!
- Add wheat germ. Add this superstar fiber booster to almost anything—soups, casseroles, meat loaf, cereals, baked goods, and so on. Wheat germ can be kept in the freezer and used without thawing. The toasted variety keeps longer than the untoasted.

9. Dress your chicken for success.   Roll skinless chicken breasts in corn bran or oat bran before baking.

10. Get into fiber sprinkles.   Top your yogurt or sorbet with bran, sunflower seeds, or chopped apples, dates, etc.

11. Make white flour a taboo.   Choose brown whole wheat when baking from scratch.

12. Drink plenty of liquids.   Fiber simply can't do its job unless you consume adequate amounts of fluid.